THE BABY BOOMERS BIBLE FOR HEALTHY BODY HEALTHY MIND

Not just another diet book — A comprehensive guide
to boomers' physical and mental fitness.
Including how to prevent diabetes, depression,
weight gain, heart problems, and dementia.

by Tracy Ayton

The Baby Boomers Bible For Healthy Body Healthy Mind

Library of Congress Cataloging-in-Publication Data

Names: Ayton, Tracy, 1964-
Title: The baby boomer's bible for healthy body healthy mind / by Tracy Ayton.
Description: Ocala, Florida : Atlantic Publishing Group, Inc., [2017] |
   Includes bibliographical references and index.
Identifiers: LCCN 2017025678 (print) | LCCN 2017025103 (ebook) | ISBN
   9781620234310 (pbk. : alk. paper) | ISBN 1620234319 (pbk. : alk. paper) |
   ISBN 9781620234327 (ebook)
Subjects: LCSH: Self-care, Health. | Nutrition. | Mind and body therapies.
Classification: LCC RA776.95 .A98 2017 (ebook) | LCC RA776.95 (print) | DDC
   613--dc23
LC record available at https://lccn.loc.gov/2017025678

Printed in the United States

PROJECT MANAGER AND EDITOR: Lisa McGinnes
COVER, JACKET & INTERIOR LAYOUT: Antoinette D'Amore • addesign@videotron.ca

Printed on Recycled Paper

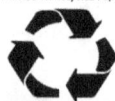

Reduce. Reuse.
RECYCLE.

A decade ago, Atlantic Publishing signed the Green Press Initiative. These guidelines promote environmentally friendly practices, such as using recycled stock and vegetable-based inks, avoiding waste, choosing energy-efficient resources, and promoting a no-pulping policy. We now use 100-percent recycled stock on all our books. The results: in one year, switching to post-consumer recycled stock saved 24 mature trees, 5,000 gallons of water, the equivalent of the total energy used for one home in a year, and the equivalent of the greenhouse gases from one car driven for a year.

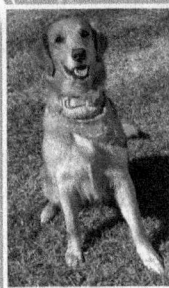

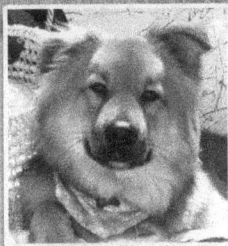

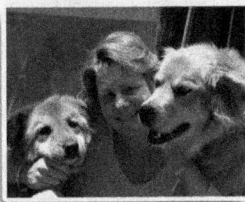

Over the years, we have adopted a number of dogs from rescues and shelters. First there was Bear and after he passed, Ginger and Scout. Now, we have Kira, another rescue. They have brought immense joy and love not just into our lives, but into the lives of all who met them.

We want you to know a portion of the profits of this book will be donated in Bear, Ginger and Scout's memory to local animal shelters, parks, conservation organizations, and other individuals and nonprofit organizations in need of assistance.

– Douglas & Sherri Brown,
President & Vice-President of Atlantic Publishing

Acknowledgments

This book and the research on which it is based would not have been possible without the help and inspiration of many people. I have gained invaluable information about nutrition and mental health during my field work, and I still get excited about the research being done for the mind and body connection and continue to further my understanding of human physiology. I am especially grateful to my editor, Lisa McGinnes, who made the publishing experience exciting and gratifying. I've appreciated the opportunity to participate in every stage as the manuscript was transformed into a book. Thank you to my husband, Richard whose unconditional love and unwavering support with an honest source of feedback and commitment. Thank you to our daughter, Aleysia, and son, Cole for your encouragement and enthusiasm and just being who you are. You both challenge me to keep reaching for the next level in life.

Table of Contents

Introduction 11

How Did I Get to Write this Book? 14

How to Use This Book 15

Chapter 1: Understanding Nutrition 17

Protein 18

Fats 22

Monounsaturated fatty acids 22

Polyunsaturated fatty acids/omega-3 (EPA and DHA) 23

Polyunsaturated fats/omega-6 (GLA and AA) 23

Saturated Fats 24

Cholesterol 24

Coconut oil 25

Trans fat 26

Fiber 26

Soluble fiber 27

Insoluble fiber 27

Water 28

Exercise and water..*28*

Carbohydrates 29

The Glycemic Index *30*

Summary...33

Chapter 2: Where Do Those Extra Pounds Come From?.............**35**

Low-Calorie Diets Don't Work 37

The Culprits 38

Sugar...*38*

White flour *39*

White rice *40*

White pasta...*41*

White potatoes...*42*

Sweet corn *42*

Leptin *43*

Summary...45

Chapter 3: The Ketogenic Diet...**47**

Forget the Calories and the Details 49

Help Food Do Its Job 49

Forget the Willpower..49

Summary...54

Chapter 4: Intermittent Fasting — Timing Your Meals **55**

How Intermittent Fasting Has
Enormous Benefits for Your Brain 59

Give Intermittent Fasting a Try 60

Summary...62

Chapter 5: Food Addiction..**63**

A Medical Condition...63

Trigger foods..*65*

Fast food...*65*

Don't worry..*65*

Set a date and stick with it *65*

Get help if you need it..*66*

Summary...66

Chapter 6: Creating the Right Mindset...................67

The Power of the Mind 67

Summary...70

Chapter 7: Diabetes...71

One of the World's Biggest Killers...................................71

The Signs and Symptoms..72

Excessive thirst and frequent urination...............................73

Intense hunger 73

Blurred vision...73

Diagnosis and Treatment 73

Stop Sugar Cravings 75

Tip #1..75

Tip #2..75

Tip #3..76

Tip #4..76

Tip #5..77

Summary...77

Chapter 8: The Brain 79

Nutrition for the Mind 80

Amino Acids: The Alphabet for Mind and Mood 81

The Jobs of Neurotransmitters 83

Tryptamine, serotonin..83

Adrenaline, noradrenaline...83

Dopamine..84

GABA (Gamma Amino Butyric Acid) 84

Acetylcholine 84

Foods That Boost Your Brain Power 85

Phospholipids...85

Pyroglutamate 87

Prostaglandins..88

Vitamins and minerals..89

Summary...91

Chapter 9: Depression and Hypoglycemia **93**

Natural Remedy 94

Sugar's Role 95

The Best Foods for People with Hypoglycemia 96

Dietary Supplements Recommended for Hypoglycemia 97

Are You Getting Enough Fat? 97

Summary 99

Chapter 10: Address Your Stress **101**

How to Counter the Stress Response 103

Get enough sleep 103

Talk to someone 106

Exercise 106

Breathe 106

Power posing 107

Adrenal Fatigue Syndrome 108

The capsule 109

The cortex 110

The medulla 110

Summary 114

Chapter 11: Reducing Your Risk of Heart Disease **115**

What is Heart Disease? 115

Preventing and Reversing Heart Disease 116

Exaggerated vs. real risk factors 117

Lower your cholesterol 117

Lower your blood pressure 118

Get your essential fats 118

Symptoms of a Heart Attack in Men 119

Symptoms of a Heart Attack in Women 120

Summary 121

Chapter 12: Dementia and Alzheimer's **123**

Quality Sleep 126

Homocysteine 127

Vitamin C 129

Summary.. 131

Chapter 13: Exercise.. 133

High-Intensity Exercise 134

Human growth hormone *135*

Telomere shortening *135*

Peak Fitness... *136*

Strength training.. *138*

Aerobic exercises *139*

Core exercises *139*

Stretching *139*

Summary.. 139

Chapter 14: Supplements 141

Multivitamin.. 141

Multimineral... 142

Vitamin C 142

Vitamin D.. 143

Vitamin K 143

Vitamin K1.. *144*

Vitamin K2.. *144*

Who needs vitamin K? *144*

Who should not take vitamin K? *145*

Amino Acids for Mind and Mood............................. 145

BCAA (branched chain amino acids)........................ *145*

Summary.. 147

**Chapter 15: Alzheimer's and Dementia Prevention
and Memory-Boosting Supplements 149**

B Vitamins 150

Astaxanthin.. 150

7-Keto-DHEA 151

DMAE 152

Phosphatidylserine (PS).. 152

Carnitine 153

Black Seed Oil: A True Panacea 154

Chapter 16: Smoking **157**

Conclusion **161**

Appendix: Recipes for the Ketogenic Diet **163**

Examples 163

Breakfast *163*

Lunch *164*

Dinner *165*

Recipes 166

Easy egg salad *166*

Meat Bagel *167*

Zucchini Chips with Smoked Paprika *168*

Zucchini Fritters *169*

Ricotta Meatball Recipe *170*

Asian Cabbage Stir-Fry *171*

Baked Salmon with Lemon and Butter *172*

Chicken Breast with Herb Butter *173*

Scrambled Eggs *174*

Mushroom Omelet *175*

Low-Carb Cauliflower Mash *176*

Broccoli and Cauliflower in Cheese *177*

Ground Beef with Red Peppers *178*

Cheeseburgers Without the Bun *179*

Fried Chicken Breast Pieces *180*

One-Pan Baked Chicken Thighs *181*

References **183**

Recommended Books **191**

Index **193**

About the Author **195**

Introduction

The baby boomers (people born between 1946 and 1964) have begun their march into old age. That's scary for most of us. It's unknown territory. Gone are the years when we would look forward to birthdays. Usually, another year would see us closer to another milestone. Like becoming a teenager at 13, learning to drive, legally sipping our first alcoholic drink, being able to vote, and celebrating our 21st with family and friends. But from the 30s onwards, anticipation gradually turns to hesitation for many adults.

In 2011, the eldest of the baby boomers turned 65. Baby boomers will more than double the number of elderly in the United States. Medical intervention has drastically extended our lifetimes by an average of

19 years. That means that about 71 million baby boomers have at least another two decades ahead of them.

We know that baby boomers are more educated and wealthier than previous generations, which should indicate improved health. But, as a group, baby boomers might need a reality check. For example, in the mid-1800s, the average man had a body mass index (BMI) of 23. In 2000, that ballooned to a BMI of 28.2. It is estimated adults aged 50–59 have the highest prevalence of obesity.

The developed world's lifestyle has shifted mainly from active to sedentary and from community-based to social isolation. Eating habits have moved from healthy, often fresh food to prepared food and takeout. This breeds depression, poor health, and chronic ailments like high blood pressure, hypertension, and diabetes.

The extra years tacked onto life expectancy should be cause for celebration, not angst. It's time to reset, make some changes, and live a life full of fun and laughter into a ripe old age starting today.

This book is to share with you what I have learned — through experience, friends, colleagues, and clients — about losing weight, living a longer and healthier life, and how we can help ourselves to prevent the onset of depression and degenerative diseases like diabetes and Alzheimer's. My philosophy as a nutritionist is to promote a holistic approach to healthy living. The complete, "Healthy Body, Healthy Mind."

First, some scary facts to motivate you.

Years of consuming too many carbohydrates, too much sugar, and not enough fat are major factors that start the brain damage cascade, coinciding with an increase in obesity, diabetes, and so many mental health issues — including depression, anxiety, and eating disorders.

Statistics are grim. Suicide, violence, and depression are on the increase. The World Health Organization says mental health is fast becoming the number one health issue this century, with one in four people suffering at some point in their lives. Mental health disorders (particularly depression) are associated with more than 90 percent of all cases of suicide. Although suicide is a genuine problem among young adults, death rates continue to be highest among older adult's ages 65 years and over. Males are four times more likely to die from suicide than females. However, females are more likely to attempt suicide than males. Studies have shown most can be prevented by a fundamental approach to diet and supplements.

As the world's waistlines have ballooned — with one in three people now overweight in the first world — so have the number of diabetes cases. Diabetes itself is the eighth biggest killer in the world. Failing to control levels of sugar in the blood has devastating health consequences. It triples the risk of a heart attack and is a leading cause of blindness, kidney failure, heart attacks, stroke, and lower limb amputation. The World Health Organization says the number of people with diabetes has risen from 108 million in 1980 to 422 million in 2014.

You can prevent, treat, and reverse diabetes, and you can certainly do something about that waistline.

One in three seniors dies with Alzheimer's or another dementia. 50 percent of 85-year-olds (the fastest growing segment of our population) will develop dementia or Alzheimer's disease. Worldwide, 47.5 million people have dementia, and there are 7.7 million new cases every year. Alzheimer's disease is the most common cause of dementia and may contribute to 60–70 percent of cases. Dementia is one of the principal causes of disability and dependency among older people worldwide. The total number of individuals with dementia is projected to be 75.6 million in 2030 and to almost triple by 2050 to 135.5 million. Women aged 60 or older are twice as likely to develop Alzheimer's as breast cancer. We need to prevent and halt the onset of Dementia and Alzheimer's.

How Did I Get to Write this Book?

When we leave home, we tend to grab everything with two hands and not worry about the consequences — Let's eat whatever we like, drink whatever we like and be merry! With absolute disregard to the ramifications of the body and the brain. Unless we have a eureka moment and adjust our food input and lifestyle, we are heading for an unhealthy, uncomfortable ,and far from merry mid/old age.

I originally worked in the beauty industry, and as I developed my business, I started coming across many clients who were dissatisfied with life. In that industry, we were also amateur psychologists; after many in-depth discussions with client's, I realized that Mind- Body-Food -Exercise links were always present. While there were often obvious external signs such as body image issues, or low self-esteem and weight issues it was clear there was more at work causing these problems. There seemed to be an epidemic of modern diseases including obesity, depression, and addictive behavior, and I realized the ramifications of lifestyle, wrong foods and over indulgence were obvious.

This was my eureka moment.

I began studying nutrition and researching these links. I developed the programs that were to eventually become this book and began working as a nutritionist. I also worked with a medical center developing a program to assist their overweight patients to deal with weight and diabetes issues. This work allowed me to show that my theories work in practice.

I was encouraged to put this information into print — hence this book.

I have aimed it at my fellow Baby Boomers as we still read books and still have time to adjust our lives and reverse the damage done. But it could just as easily be the Mid Life Guide to Healthy Body Healthy Mind. Its aim is to help you reach that eureka moment and make the adjustments to improve all aspects of your life and work on preventing what are often described as age related diseases that are more than likely caused by your lifestyle. I believe you can eat your way to a healthier life.

What we eat has a dramatic effect on our body and mind. My mission is help as many people on their journey to become 100% healthy without medication. Eating the right foods can help you achieve and maintain a healthy weight that can be maintained. Try to check health markers before you start your lifestyle change — markers like blood sugar (fasting blood glucose and HbA1c), blood pressure, and your cholesterol profile (including HDL, triglycerides). These are universally used. Re-evaluating these health markers after a couple of months can be great a great motivational tool — they'll usually show that not only are you losing weight, but you're improving your health too.

How to Use This Book

Like all nonfiction authors, I have had to juggle between telling a good story and presenting the facts. One of my friends says not to let the facts get in the way of a good story, but if we are going to understand how our bodies work, we need the correct information.

As a result, you will come across many unpronounceable names. Scientists, like attorneys and doctors, seem to prefer a language only they can understand. I apologize in advance, but it's necessary to get the story right.

All the parts of this book fit together to give a complete guide. But, like the Bible, they can be read separately (perhaps just one part in a sitting) so you can take it all in.

The body is an incredibly complicated machine. To make maximum use of the information, you need to understand each part of the book. You don't have to read it in any order; you can go straight to the section that interests you. But as most functions of the body are interlinked, you need to read it all to fully understand what you need to do to improve your life.

Here we go — good luck.

Chapter 1

Understanding Nutrition

We are not only physically what we eat, but how we think and feel is directly affected by what we eat and drink. Do you oscillate between feeling good and feeling like crap (FLC syndrome)?

How balanced is your mood? Your thinking, feeling, mental energy, and focus happen across a network of interconnecting brain cells, each of which depends on an optimal supply of nutrients to work efficiently. So, guess what? You can and will change how you think and feel by what you put in your mouth!

A fundamentally new approach to wellbeing is a must. We must empower ourselves to become healthy, vibrant, motivated, and happy. Time to get our mojo back and look and feel fabulous. Healthy body, healthy mind.

Good nutrition is the foundation of good health. Everyone needs the five basic nutrients — protein, carbohydrates, fats, fiber, and water — as well as vitamins, minerals, and other micronutrients. To better understand why those foods should be supported with supplements, you need to have a clear idea of the components of a healthy diet.

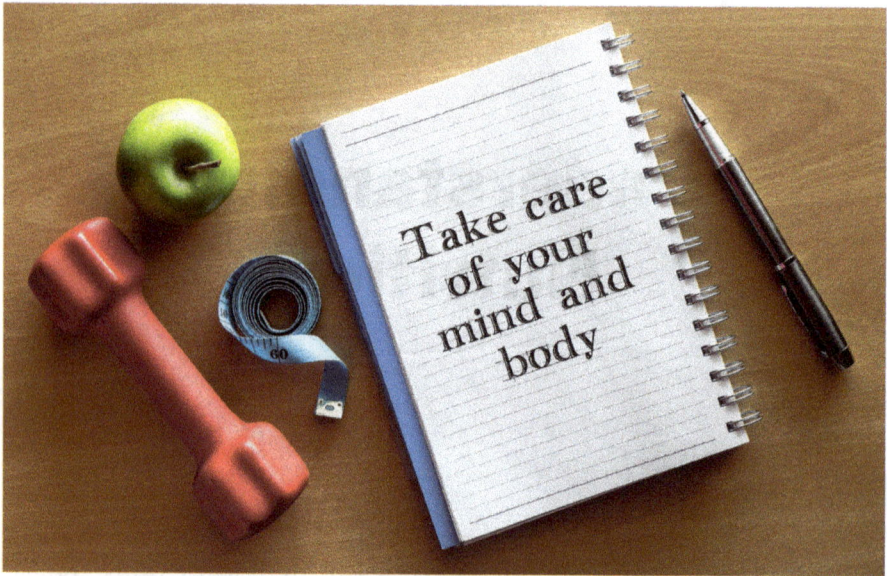

Protein

Protein is essential for growth and development. It is the building block of body tissue and can also serve as a fuel source for muscles, organs, the brain, and the skeletal structure. When protein is consumed, the body breaks it down into simpler bodies called amino acids. Some amino acids are produced by the body, but for the most part, they are introduced into the system through ingesting different foods. There are nine essential amino acids which humans must obtain from their diet to prevent protein-energy malnutrition. These are phenylalanine, valine, threonine, tryptophan, methionine, leucine, isoleucine, lysine, and histidine. And there are five dispensable amino acids which humans can synthesize in the body: alanine, aspartic acid, asparagine, glutamic acid, and serine.

Humans need the essential amino acids in certain ratios. Some protein sources contain amino acids in a more or less "complete" sense. This has given rise to various ranking systems for protein sources. A complete protein is a source of protein that contains an adequate proportion of the nine essential amino acids necessary for the dietary needs. Proteins derived from animal foods are complete [poultry, fish, eggs, milk, cheese, yogurt].

Incomplete proteins are those that don't contain all nine essential amino acids, or don't have sufficient quantities of them to meet the body's needs, [vegetables, fruits, oats, seeds and nuts] and must be supplemented with other proteins. Just because they are incomplete doesn't make them inferior, though; they just need to be combined to provide the right balance of essential aminos. Proteins that, in combination, make a complete amino acid profile are known as complementary proteins. Here are a few tasty examples: Spinach salad with almonds, beef patties with vegetables, venison meatballs with peanut sauce, three egg omelettes with onions.

Protein is a nutrient needed by the human body for maintenance and growth. Proteins are the most abundant kind of molecules in the body, aside from water. Protein can be found in all cells of the body and is the major structural component of all cells in the body, especially muscle. This also includes body organs, hair, and skin.

Considerable debate has taken place regarding issues surrounding protein intake requirements. The amount of protein required in a person's diet is determined in large part by overall energy intake, the body's need for nitrogen and essential amino acids, body weight and composition, rate of growth in the individual, physical activity level, individual's energy and carbohydrate intake, as well as the presence of illness or injury. Physical activity and exertion, as well as enhanced muscle mass, increase the need for protein. Requirements are also greater during childhood for growth and development, during pregnancy or when breastfeeding to nourish a baby, or when the body needs to recover from malnutrition, trauma, or an operation. Protein comes from two sources:

- Animal sources, such as meats, fish, cheese, eggs, and milk.
- Vegetable Sources, such as soybeans, almonds, hazelnuts, peanuts, and legumes.

A diet low in protein can lead to serious problems like muscle deterioration, wrinkling of the skin, and immune deficiencies. Later on, we will see how supplementing amino acids can solve many mental health issues. But just eating complete proteins daily you will improve your mind and your emotions.

If the amount of protein consumed is too high, when physical exercise is low, unburned protein residues will remain in the body and be converted into uric acid, which can lead to gout. So, how much protein do we need to eat? It depends on your age.

	Age (Years)	RDI Protein (ounces/day)
Infants/Toddlers	1-3	0.4oz
Children	4-8	0.7oz
Boys	9-13	1.4oz

	Age (Years)	RDI Protein (ounces/day)
	14-18	2.3oz
Girls	9-13	1.2oz
	14-18	1.5oz
Men	19-70	2.2oz
	70	2.8oz
Women	19-70	1.6oz
	70	2oz
Pregnancy	14-18	2.01oz
	19-50	2.1oz
Breastfeeding	14-50	2.3oz

RDI = Recommended Daily Intake

Here are some examples of protein content of foods, in ounces.

One grilled lean beef fillet steak (4.7oz. weight)	1.2oz protein
One grilled chicken breast (3.7oz. weight)	1.1oz protein
1/2 baked fillet snapper (4.3oz. weight)	0.9oz protein
One can tuna in spring water (3.5oz weight)	0.89oz protein
One grilled pork leg steak (2.8oz weight)	0.6oz protein

1/4 can boiled red kidney beans (3.5oz weight)	0.2oz protein
Tofu (3.5oz weight)	0.28oz protein
1 cup trim milk (8.8oz weight)	0.35oz protein
One boiled egg (1.7oz weight)	0.21oz protein
One tub plain, low-fat yogurt (5.2oz weight)	0.25oz protein
1/4 can baked beans in tomato sauce (3.5oz weight)	0.17oz protein
One slice multigrain bread (1.4oz weight)	0.18oz protein
One slice white bread (1.5oz weight)	0.10 protein
Ten almonds (0.4oz weight)	0.08oz protein
2cm cube Edam cheese (0.2oz weight)	0.07oz protein

Fats

There are numerous types of fat. Fat is essential for your health because it supports some your body's functions. Some vitamins, for instance, must have fat to be absorbed and for your body use them. Essential fats reduce the risk of cancer, allergies, fatigue, depression, PMS, and Alzheimer's disease.

Monounsaturated fatty acids

Studies show that consuming foods rich in monounsaturated fatty acids can improve blood cholesterol levels, which can reduce your risk of heart disease. Research also shows that these fatty acids may benefit blood sugar control and insulin levels — especially helpful if you have type 2 diabetes. Examples of foods high in monounsaturated fats include plant-based liquid oils such as olive oil, peanut oil, canola oil, sesame oil, and safflower oil. Other sources include peanut butter, avocados, and many nuts and seeds.

Polyunsaturated fatty acids/omega-3 (EPA and DHA)

It's from these fats that our body and brain make prostaglandins, an essential hormone-like substance that helps lower blood pressure, boosts immunity, and decreases inflammation. Studies show that by eating foods rich in polyunsaturated fatty acids improves blood cholesterol levels, which can decrease your risk of heart disease. These fatty acids may also help lower the possibility of type 2 diabetes.

Foods high in omega-3 fats come from plant-based oils, including corn oil, soybean oil, and sunflower oil (that are liquid at room temperature), and fatty fish such as mackerel, salmon, trout, and herring. Some nuts and seeds such as sunflower seeds and walnuts, soybeans, and tofu are also high in omega-3 fats.

Polyunsaturated fats/omega-6 (GLA and AA)

The brain has the highest portion of omega-6 than any other tissue in the body. Omega-6 plays an important role in cell growth and is thus essential for brain and muscle development. The omega-6 arachidonic acid (AA) is for this very reason added to most infant formulas. Both brain development and muscle development are critical for infants. The growth benefits of omega-6 also explain the great interest that body-builders and top athletes have in omega-6 consumption. Omega-6 in the form of linoleic acid (LA) plays a critical role in the production of hormone-like messengers. These PGE1 messengers from LA trigger immune responses, reduce fluid accumulation, and impact depression, multiple sclerosis, PMS mood swings, schizophrenia, ADHD (attention deficit hyperactivity disorder), and other brain disorders.

Messengers made from arachidonic acid (AA) are called PGE2 and play an important role in swelling, pain, blood thinning, blood vessel spasms, and accumulation of inflamed cells. You may wonder why pain or inflammation is considered a benefit. The answer is that pain is an important signal that prevents further injury, and inflammation is a trigger for our immune system.

Two common omega-6 acids are linoleic acid and arachidonic acid. Linoleic acid can be found in abundance in corn oil, soybean, safflower, and sunflower oils. And arachidonic acid, or AA, is found in large quantities in dairy and animal meats and fats.

Saturated Fats

Saturated fats occur naturally in many foods. The majority come mainly from animal sources, including meat and dairy products. Examples of foods containing saturated fats are lamb, fatty beef, pork, chicken with skin, lard and cream, beef fat, butter, and cheese and other dairy products made with whole milk. The most important thing to remember is the overall dietary picture. Saturated fats are just one piece of the puzzle. In general, you can't go wrong eating more polyunsaturated and monounsaturated fats and vegetables.

Cholesterol

We all need some cholesterol to help our brains, skin, and other organs grow and do their jobs in the body. Cholesterol is an important biological chemical — maybe the most important in the body. It serves as a parent compound to numerous skin moisture factors. It is a crucial component of the membrane that surrounds each of the estimated 100 trillion cells in the body, where it is used as a precursor to dozens of essential biochemical substances including cortisol, vitamin D, DHEA, progesterone, estrogen, testosterone, and many other reproductive hormones. There are two types of cholesterol — low-density lipoprotein and high-density liporprotein.

LDL cholesterol is more likely to clog blood vessels because it carries the cholesterol away from the liver into the bloodstream, where it can stick to the blood vessels. HDL cholesterol, on the other hand, carries the cholesterol back to the liver where it is broken down.

Here's a way to remember the difference. LDL cholesterol is the bad kind, so call it "lousy" cholesterol — "L" for lousy. The HDL is the good cholesterol, so remember it as "healthy" cholesterol — "H" for healthy.

Coconut oil

Some plant-based oils, such as coconut oil, contain a lot of saturated fats. There is a misconception that coconut oil is not good for heart health. This is because it contains a lot of saturated fats. In reality, it is super beneficial for the heart. It contains about 50 percent lauric acid, which helps in actively preventing various heart problems like high cholesterol levels and high blood pressure. Coconut oil does not lead to increase in LDL levels, and it reduces the incidence of injury and damage to arteries and therefore helps in preventing atherosclerosis.

Research suggests that intake of coconut oil may help to maintain healthy lipid profiles in premenopausal women. Research also suggests that coconut oil contributes to reducing abdominal obesity in women. It is also easy to digest, and it helps in healthy functioning of the thyroid and endocrine system. Further, it increases the body's metabolic rate by removing stress on the pancreas, thereby burning more energy and helping obese and overweight people lose the weight. People living in tropical coastal areas who use coconut oil every day as their primary cooking oil are normally not obese or overweight.

Trans fat

This is a type of fat occurs naturally in some foods in small amounts, but most trans fats are made from oils through a food processing called partial hydrogenation. These are the fats to be avoided, as they are partially hydrogenated trans fats that can increase unhealthy LDL cholesterol and lower good HDL cholesterol. This can increase your risk of cardiovascular disease.

Trans fats are easy to use, inexpensive to produce, and last a long time. Trans fats give foods a desirable taste and texture. Many restaurants and fast-food outlets use trans fats to deep-fry foods because oils with trans fats can be used many times in commercial fryers. Trans fats can be found in many foods like donuts, pie crusts, biscuits, frozen pizza, crackers, and cookies. You should consume less than two grams of trans fat per day. Read the nutritional labels.

Fiber

Fiber is a substance found mainly in vegetables, fruit, and whole cereals. It has no energy value but plays a significant role in the digestive process. The cellulose, pectin, lignin, and the gums they contain ensure good intestinal function, and their absence is the cause of most constipation.

Research shows that people who eat more fiber tend to be leaner and are less likely to gain weight over time. There are two major categories of fiber — soluble and insoluble. Both play a key role in preventing disease and promoting health. Foods containing fiber make you feel fuller after you eat it. That's because when a meal contains fiber, the food moves more slowly from your stomach into your small intestine. For example, if you eat a meal that contains 300 calories and 10 grams of fiber, you will feel more satisfied (and stay satisfied longer) than if you eat a meal with same number calories but no fiber.

Fiber does some other beneficial things as well, depending on whether it is soluble or insoluble.

Soluble fiber

If you stir some soluble fiber into hot water, it will dissolve. In your stomach, the soluble fiber you've eaten dissolves in the water from your food and digestive juices to make a viscous liquid or gel. This gel can trap individual food components and make them less available for absorption. Soluble fiber's fat binding action can help reduce cholesterol. And by slowing down the absorption of sugar, it helps keep blood sugar levels steadier — which is helpful for managing and preventing diabetes. Most fruits and vegetables also provide soluble fiber. Psyllium husks, which are very high in soluble fiber, are very popular.

Insoluble fiber

Insoluble fiber won't dissolve if stirred into hot water. As soon as you stop stirring, it'll just sink to the bottom. However, it will soak up water and expand the way a dry sponge expands as it soaks up water. Now, imagine this expanded sponge moving through your intestines and you will begin to get an idea of how insoluble fiber works. It is a very effective treatment and preventative for constipation and other digestive disorders like diverticulitis and irritable bowel syndrome.

Water

How much water does our body require? The human body is about 60 percent water. We're always losing water from our bodies via urine and sweat. There are many different opinions on how much water we should be drinking every day. Health authorities commonly recommend eight 8-ounce glasses, which equals about 2 liters, or half a gallon. This is called the 8×8 rule and is very easy to remember.

However, other health experts think we're always on the brink of dehydration and that we need to sip on water regularly throughout the day, even when we're not thirsty. As with most things, this depends on the individual, and there are many factors (both internal and external) that ultimately affect our need for water. Lack of fluids can lead to dehydration, a condition that occurs when you don't have enough water in your body to carry out normal functions. Even mild dehydration can drain your energy and make you tired. You may need to modify your total fluid intake depending on how active you are, the climate you live in, your health status, and if you're pregnant or breastfeeding.

Exercise and water

If you are exercising or are engaging in activities that make you sweat, you will need to drink extra water to compensate for the fluid loss. An extra 15 to 20 ounces (2 glasses) of water should be sufficient for short bursts of exercise, but intense exercise lasting for more than an hour requires more fluid intake. How much additional fluid you need depends on how much you sweat during exercise and the duration and type of exercise.

During long bouts of intense exercise, it's best to use a sports drink that contains sodium, as this will help replace sodium lost in sweat. Also, continue to replace fluids after you've finished exercising.

The environment can also have an effect. Humid or hot weather can make you sweat and requires an additional intake of fluid. Illnesses or health conditions can have an effect as well, especially when you have a fever, are vomiting, or have diarrhea. In these cases, your body loses additional fluids and you should drink more water.

Women who are pregnant or breastfeeding need additional fluids to stay hydrated. Significant amounts of fluid are used during nursing. Water is your best bet because it's readily available, calorie free, and not expensive. But you do not need to rely only on what you drink to meet your fluid needs.

What you eat also provides a sizable portion of your fluid needs. On average, food provides about 20 percent of total water intake. For example, many fruits and vegetables, such as watermelon and spinach, are 90 percent or more water by weight. Also, beverages such as milk and juice are composed mostly of water. Even caffeinated beverages — such as coffee, tea or soda — can contribute. But these should not be a major portion of your daily total fluid intake because of the caffeine and calories.

Carbohydrates

There are so many misconceptions and preconceived ideas about carbohydrates. I am going to discuss this at some length because it is this food group that causes us to store fat. For many years, carbohydrates were placed into two distinct categories. Quick sugars — simple sugars such as cane sugar, honey, and fruit. Or slow sugars — more complex molecules such as starches and cereals. This way of classifying carbohydrates is completely outdated and is based on an incorrect theory.

Carbohydrates are molecules composed of carbon, oxygen, and hydrogen. To illustrate, let's look at a tree. An apple tree. The roots absorb hydrogen and oxygen from the soil, water and absorb carbon and oxygen from the air, carbon dioxide. The sun penetrates the plant and together these atoms form carbohydrates (COH). This is a carbohydrate in its purest form. You eat the apple; the body breaks it down into glucose. Glucose is the body's principle fuel. It is stored in the form of glycogen in the muscles and liver. Glycaemia is the term used here for the level of glucose in the bloodstream. On an empty stomach, this glucose level is usually one gram per liter of blood. When carbohydrate has been ingested on an empty stomach, the effect on the blood sugar level is as follows.

In the first phase, glycemia rises (to a degree, according to the nature of the carbohydrate). In the second phase, following secretion of insulin from the pancreas, the blood glucose level falls, and the glucose is released into the body's tissues. In the third phase, blood sugar levels revert to normal. So, what matters is to consider the effect of different carbohydrates on the glycemic level — in other words, how much glucose they produce. This is called the glycemic index.

The Glycemic Index

The glycemic index (GI) is a ranking of carbohydrates on a scale from 0 to 100 according to the extent to which they raise blood sugar levels after eating. Foods with a high GI are those which are rapidly digested and absorbed and result in marked fluctuations in blood sugar levels. Low-GI foods, by their slow digestion and absorption, produce gradual rises in blood sugar and insulin levels and have proven benefits for health. Low GI diets have been shown to improve both glucose and lipid levels in people with diabetes (type 1 and type 2). They have benefits for weight control because they help control appetite and delay hunger. Low GI diets also reduce insulin levels and insulin resistance.

Insulin is the fat hormone secreted by the pancreas that plays a vital role in our metabolism. How much insulin is secreted by the pancreas depends on what carbohydrate you consume. Carbohydrates are broken down by the body into glucose. The pancreas secretes insulin, and it is insulin's role to move that glucose through the body for immediate energy. What the body doesn't use for immediate energy gets stored in the muscle for future use. When the muscle is full, the glucose gets stored in the liver for future use, and when the liver is full it immediately gets stored as fat! As I said above, how much glucose is stored away in the form of fat depends on the type of carbohydrate consumed.

Unfortunately, the way many of us have eaten over the last few decades has made this process a fat storage unit. Too much insulin, too much fat! Control insulin, lose weight. We completely overload blood glucose by the foods we are eating.

We have a food industry that is killing us. There is so much over-processed food on store shelves, mainly devoid of anything nutritious, that often we don't even recognize what we are eating. How many times have you picked up a package to look at the ingredients and been unable to pronounce the word, let alone recognize what it is? Seriously! But because the picture on the cover looks so delicious, we take it home. The food industry pays big dollars to food scientists to make their foods addictive. Diets that center mainly around packaged food, frozen food, and fast food are probably contributing to this nutrition disaster.

See the chart below for examples of GI. Foods under 50 on the GI do not affect blood sugar or insulin. .

Low Glycemic Foods List 0-55	Medium Glycemic Foods List 56-70	High Glycemic Foods List 70+
Most non starchy vegetable <15	Canned kidney beans 52	Bagel 72
Peanuts <15	Kiwifruit 52	Corn chips 72
Low-fat yogurt, no sugar <15	Orange juice 52	Watermelon 72
Tomatoes 15	Banana 53	Honey 73
Cherries 22	Potato chips 54	Mashed potatoes 73
Peas 22	Special K 54	Cheerios 74
Plum 24	Sweet potato 54	Puffed wheat 74
Grapefuit 25	Brown Rice 54	Doughnuts 75
Pearled barley 25	Linguine 55	French fries 76
Peach 28	Oatmeal cookies 55	Vanilla wafers 77
Can peaches, natural juice 30	Popcorn 55	White bread 79
Soy milk 30	Muesli 5	Jelly beans 80
Baby lima beans 32	White rice 56	Pretzels 81
Fat-free milk 32	Pita bread 57	Rice cakes 82
Low-fat yogurt, with sugar 33	Blueberry muffin 59	Mashed potatoes, instant 83
Apple 36	Bran muffin 60	Cornflakes 84
Pear 36	Hamburger bun 61	Baked potato 85
Whole wheat spaghetti 37	Ice cream 61	Rice, instant 91
Tomato soup 38	Canned apricots, light syrup 64	French bread 95
Carrots, cooked 39	Macaroni and cheese 64	Parsnips 97
Apple juice 41	Raisins 64	Dates 100
All-Bran 42	Couscous 65	
Canned chickpeas 42	Quick-cooking porridge 65	
	Rye crisp-bread 65	

Low Glycemic Foods List 0-55	Medium Glycemic Foods List 56-70	High Glycemic Foods List 70+
Custard 43	Table sugar (sucrose) 65	
Grapes 43	Instant porridge 66	
Orange 43	Pineapple 66	
Canned lentil soup 44	Taco shells 68	
Macaroni 45	Whole wheat bread 68	
Pineapple juice 46		
Banana bread 47		
Long-grain rice 47		
Bulgur 48		
Canned baked beans 48		
Grapefuit juice 48		
Green peas 48		
Oat bran bread 48		
Old-fashioned porridge 49		Compiled by: www.LowGIHealth.com.au from various sources

Summary

Remember, we are not only physically what we eat, but how we think and feel is directly affected by what we eat and drink. Good nutrition is the foundation of good health. Everyone needs the five basic nutrients — protein, carbohydrates, fats, fiber, and water — as well as vitamins, minerals, and other micronutrients.

Eat more eggs, chicken, seafood, and shellfish — all of which contain important protein and amino acids and are extremely rich in both

DHA and AA (essential omegas). Eat more fats. Essential fats reduce the risk of cancer, allergies, fatigue, depression, PMS, and Alzheimer's disease. Choose olive oil for cooking and salad dressing due to its high omega-3 content.

The glycemic index is for everybody — including those with diabetes. Reduce carbohydrate consumption. The glycemic index (GI) is a ranking of carbohydrates on a scale from 0 to 100 according to the extent to which they raise blood sugar levels after eating. Low GI foods result in slow and sustained release of glucose in the blood, so these are the best food for most people.

Chapter 2

Where Do Those Extra Pounds Come From?

Let's look closer at where those extra pounds come from.

My dieting days began in my late 20s when I became a devotee to the culinary delights available, coupled with sublime New Zealand Sauvignon Blancs and Chardonnays. The combination of these new foods and wine became a wake-up call for my 27-year-old dormant fat cells. And boy did they party! The weight piled on staggeringly quick. So, my days of ridiculous diets and deprivation — thrown in with pills, lotions, and potions — began.

My first diet was cabbage soup. Can you imagine eating nothing but cabbage soup for ten days, then a rather limited monotonous diet for another two weeks? It was an easy diet if you never left the house and slept all the time!

Yes, I lost weight, but I almost lost the will to live. Virtually any kind of absurd diet can lead to weight loss. Most fad diets fail in the long run because of the monotony and deprivation imposed. When you lose weight quickly, you put it back on just as quickly. Little did I know that I had just triggered an ancestral survival mechanism for periods of famine, which make the body go into fat storage mode. My body responded by converting and storing every morsel of food into fat, and so my days of weight loss, weight gain, weight loss, and weight gain started. We need to wake up and stop the yoyo dieting forever!

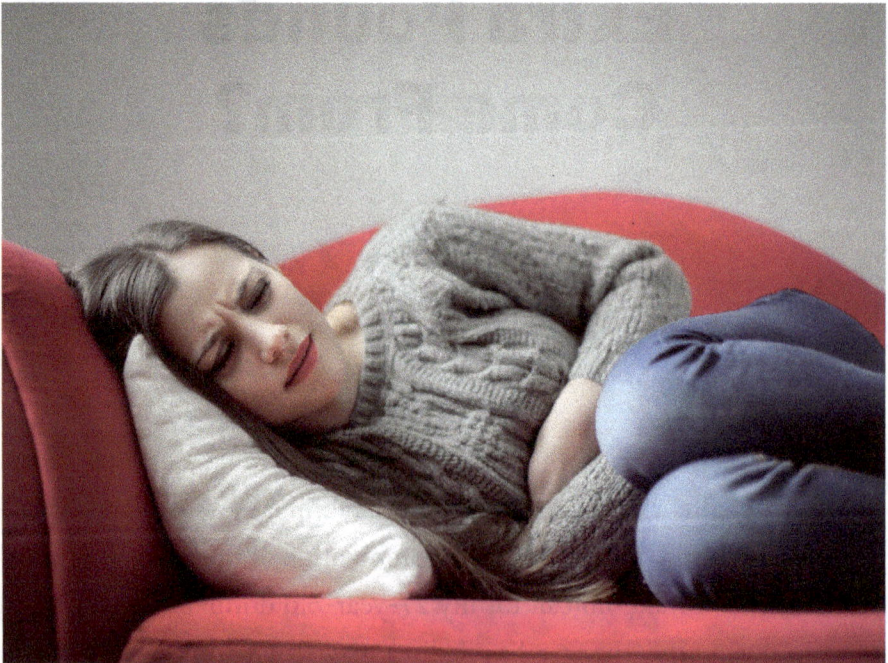

Low-Calorie Diets Don't Work

In the short term, low-calorie diets can be marginally successful, but in the long run, they make the problem worse. Humans, like animals, have sophisticated biological systems to protect them from periods of starvation, common when our hunter-gatherer ancestors were unable to find enough food. Whenever there is a decrease in calorie consumption — in other words, when you eat less than you need for basic biological function — your body throws the brakes on your metabolism. Restricting calorie intake leads to other negative consequences. Immune function and adrenal gland activity reduce, and the body becomes malnourished. The lack of fiber, vitamins, minerals, amino acids, and essential fatty acids also leads to poor health.

There's also the added complication of muscle wasting. Low-calorie diets result in some degree of muscle wasting. Apart from the undesirable appearance, muscle mass is a major factor in the burning of calories. So, by losing muscle mass, your ability to burn calories will be further diminished. These responses to calorie restriction are just some of the mechanisms involved in the disastrous long-term effects of low-calorie dieting.

Globally, calorie consumption in Western countries is from 30 to 35 percent lower than 50 years ago. Paradoxically, obesity has risen by 400 percent during the same time lapse in these countries. In France, there are four times more obese people now than in the 1960s. Particularly noticeable was research done in Russia, which found that 56 percent of the women over 30 are obese and do not consume more than 1500 calories a day for a daily workload that typically demands enormous energy expenditure. This is below the daily recommended energy intake.

Similar findings were found when Professor Creff published statistics on the medical check-ups of obese people in the hospital where he worked, the Hospital Saint-Michel in Paris. He observed that over 50 percent of the people who are obese eat very little.

The Culprits

Sugar

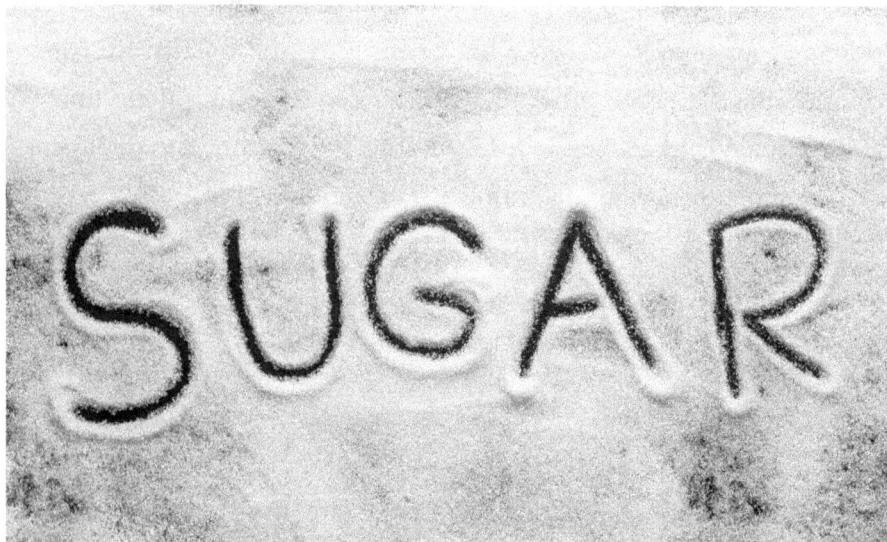

Number one on the list is fittingly the No. 1 culprit for weight gain — sugar. Sugar is poison. It saturates our bloodstream with glucose, therefore raising a massive amount of insulin to cope with the flood of blood glucose and then going on to cause insulin resistance, diabetes, and obesity.

Sugar is one of the most addictive and harmful substances we are consuming. An astounding study showed that 94 percent of rats who were given a choice between cocaine and sugar water chose the sugar. Even rats who were already addicted to cocaine quickly switched their preference to sugar once sugar was offered as a choice. The rats were also far more eager to work for sugar than for cocaine, sometimes becoming quite vicious against other rats. The researchers speculate that our sweet receptors (two protein receptors located on the tongue which evolved in ancestral times when the diet was very low in sugar) have not adapted to modern high sugar consumption.

Therefore, the abnormally high stimulation of these receptors by our sugar-rich diets generates excessive reward signals in the brain, which have the potential to override normal self-control mechanisms and lead to addiction. Refined sugar was almost non-existent in the diet of most people until very recently. Today, the overconsumption of sugar not only contributes to but drives the current obesity epidemic.

Reducing your sugar intake should be on the top of your to-do list, regardless of whether you're currently overweight or not. Why? Because it has been proven over and over that sugar increases your insulin levels, which can lead to high cholesterol and high blood pressure, diabetes, heart disease, weight gain, depression, and premature aging.

White flour

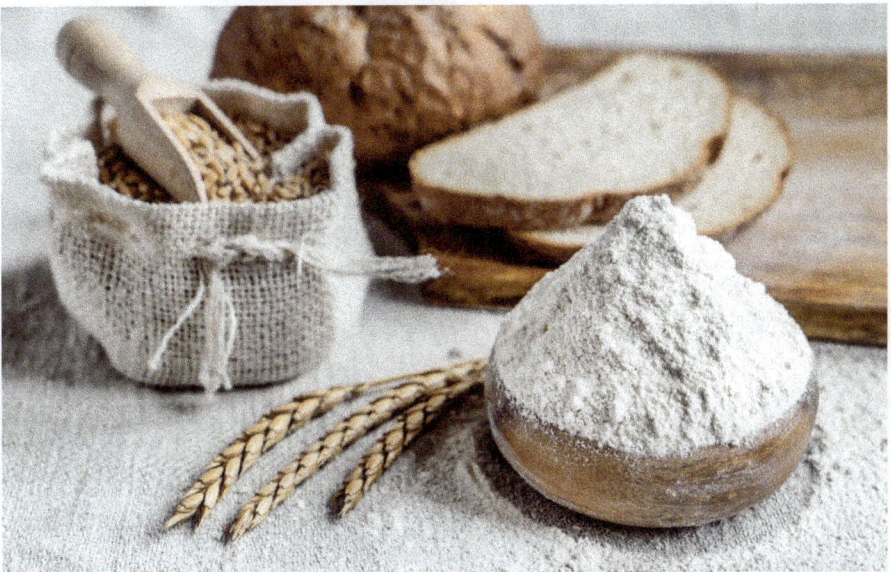

White flour is another food entirely devoid of anything nutritious, as it's been processed and bleached. White flour is the root of many problems with blood glucose because it gets broken down into glucose just about as quickly as sugar, therefore raising insulin levels and fat storage. White flour is wheat that has been stripped of two main components — the germ and the bran. The bran provides the fiber that is often found in the whole grain, but when it is processed out of white flour, it creates a lighter, softer texture. That is why whole-wheat flour is denser and heavier. That's the fiber and the added weight of the other components missing from white flour. The trouble is, the light and airy texture of white bread is devoid of its nutritional quality.

White rice

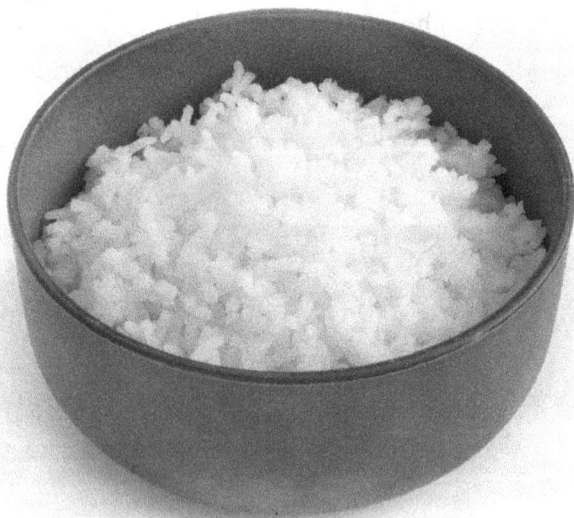

White rice is the name given to milled rice that has had its husk, bran, and germ removed. This alters the flavor, texture, and appearance of the rice and helps prevent spoilage and extend its storage life. After milling, the rice is polished, resulting in a seed with a bright, white, shiny appearance. The milling and polishing processes both remove important nutrients, so white rice is devoid of nutrition and therefore causes an insulin spike, much like flour.

White pasta

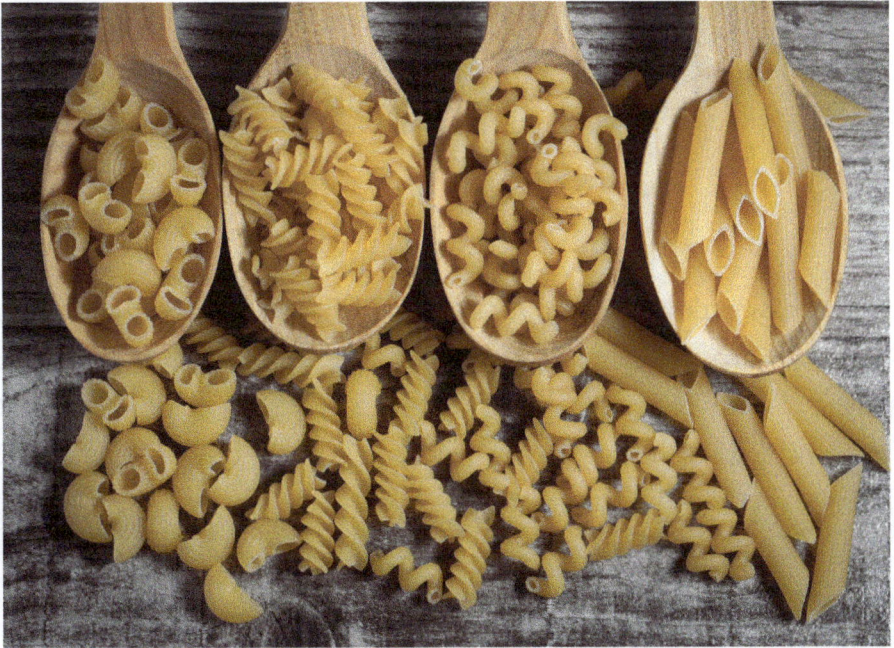

White pasta is made from refined wheat and white flour and has been milled to remove the bran and germ from the kernel. Refined wheat and white flour are made by grinding up only the endosperm portion of the grain. The process of refining gives the flour a finer texture and longer shelf life but also results in lower amounts of some beneficial nutrients. So, once again, the same zero nutritional value as white flour, and it should be avoided!

White potatoes

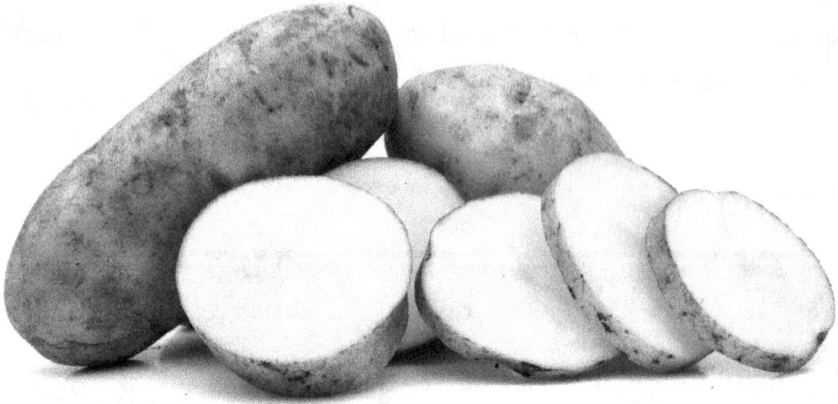

Because potatoes are comprised of more than 92 percent carbohydrates (in the form of sugar and starch), they are relatively high on the glycemic index scale. The glycemic index rates foods on a scale of 1 to 100 based on how quickly they raise your blood sugar levels. Foods closer to 100 elevate your blood sugar faster than foods on the lower end of the scale. Mashed potatoes and boiled white potatoes are 82 and 87 on the glycemic scale, respectively. Not a good food source.

Sweet corn

Experts have termed carbohydrates that raise blood sugar levels rapidly as "bad carbs." The rapid rise in blood sugar causes excessive insulin production, which may result in increased body fat. These carbohydrates are therefore more likely to cause obesity, and sweet corn is one of them. Did you know that farmers feed corn to cattle to fatten them up? We need to take action!

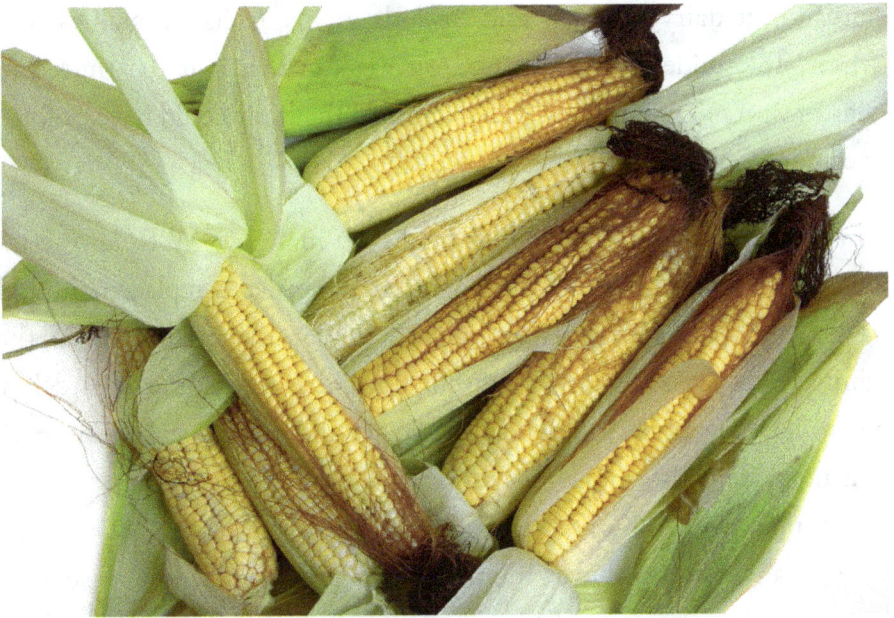

Leptin

Finally, we come to the gatekeeper of fat metabolism. Leptin is the satisfaction hormone produced by fat cells. It sends messages to the hypothalamus in the brain to say, "Ok, we have enough fat stored. Increase metabolism and decrease hunger." Unfortunately, we are consuming food that disrupts this message, thus causing havoc in our bodies. It's called high fructose corn syrup (HFCS), also known as glucose-fructose syrup or maize syrup. It is an ingredient that has glucose converted into fructose to enhance its sweetness. It's in almost every processed food that requires a sweetener, and it's in most beverages as well. You will find it in everything from bread to soup to soda.

At the time the low-fat dietary guidelines were conceived, people thought that saturated fat was a significant cause of heart disease. This is the reason the large health organizations moved away from meat, eggs, and full-fat dairy products and towards grains, fruits, vegetables, and wheat. The guidelines were based on weak evidence at the time, and many respected scientists objected and said that they could have unforeseen consequences.

The low-fat guidelines were first published in 1977. With all the fat taken out, food tasted like cardboard! They needed a replacement and fast. Sugar was too expensive to replace the fat. During the 1970s, the United States was in a lot of domestic turmoil. It was a time of hardship, with many remembering the fuel shortages and rationing that occurred, but there were also problems with cane sugar coming into the country. With political revolutions happening in sugar producing nations, climate changes creating, even more, sugar shortages, and a free trade market regulating the price of the commodity, the average person couldn't afford real sugar.

This shortage caused everyone to begin looking for alternatives, and people remembered that you could create sugars from starchy products. What food had a lot of starch with a lot of by-products? Corn. This is where high fructose corn syrup came into its own. With so much waste involved in the processing of corn, they discovered that a by-product of corn was a useful sweetener. It was much, much sweeter than sugar, had the consistency of fat, and was cheap to produce. So, fat was replaced by this natural sweetener and therefore considered healthy.

Little did we know they were setting the globe up for an epidemic of obesity, diabetes, heart disease, and mental health issues. The body did not recognize this food. Our body can convert sugar into glucose, but this is fructose. Our bodies don't recognize fructose the same way. It has to get it out of the blood stream, and the quickest way is straight to the liver, where it is stored as fat. With fructose, fat stores increase at levels the body can't cope with, interfering with the communication between leptin and the hypothalamus to say, "Enough fat, stop eating." The hypo-thalamus then presumes the body isn't producing leptin and must be starving, so it decreases metabolism and increases hunger.

The result? We get fatter and hungrier. We are now in the midst of a global pandemic of obesity, metabolic syndrome, and type 2 diabetes. The war on saturated fat is the biggest mistake in the history of nutrition.

Summary

Low-calorie diets don't work. It's what we eat that matters. Reducing certain foods is imperative.

First on the list is sugar — it's poison! Reducing your sugar intake should be on the top of your to-do list, regardless of whether you're currently overweight or not. Why? Because it has been proven over and over that sugar increases your insulin levels, which can lead to high cholesterol and high blood pressure, diabetes, heart disease, weight gain, depression and premature aging. Also reduce white flour, white rice, white pasta, sweetcorn, and potatoes. Read food labels and don't consume foods that contain leptin (HFCS) which all increase your insulin levels.

Low-calorie diets don't work. It's what you eat that will help you lose weight and keep it off. That's how we got overweight. Now for some answers.

Chapter 3

The Ketogenic Diet

Finally, a diet that controls hunger, is pleasing to the palate, provides all the necessary nutrients required by the body and brain, and is satisfying.

Real, whole, delicious, and nutritious food. It's our ancestral way of eating that encourages weight loss, boosts energy levels, and reduces the risk of diabetes, heart disease, cancer, and chronic illness. Our hunter-gatherer ancestors would have had a diet less complicated yet highly nutritious — focusing mainly on meats, chicken, seafood, and shellfish. All of which are extremely rich in both DHA and AA (essential omegas).

Upon making a kill, the Homo sapiens in East Africa wasted nothing. They consumed the whole animal. The meat was completely removed. Bones were stripped of marrow and crushed to get every bit. Offal and fat were eaten. Heads were prized for essential fatty, nutrient-rich, energy-dense food. Eating the whole animal is the kind of consumption our body can adapt to. Diverging from that diet has created many of our problems.

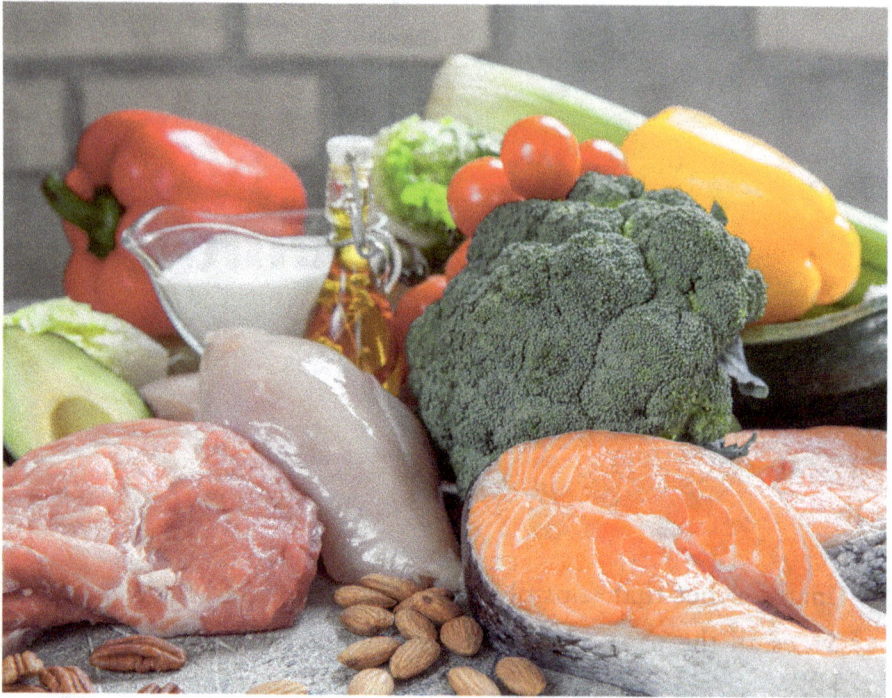

Our ancestors did not eat processed foods or pop a frozen dinner into the microwave. If your food comes in a bag, box. or package, it probably isn't real food. Your hard-earned money should not be profiting companies that produce foods full of salt, sugar, and fats to make it tasty. Just imagine what it's doing to the body. Dump the junk!

Forget the Calories and the Details

Move towards food quality. Improve the connections between you and your loved ones as you share meals. Improve the connection between you and your land as you grow, pick, and process your food. Value your tradition and history. No matter how big or small your food budget, make sure you get your money's worth. Food is fuel for your body. Food should nourish us. Does your food nourish your body? Nourish your soul? Nourish your life? Does your food sustain your heritage and tradition?

Help Food Do Its Job

Eat a broad range of foods. Eat real food. Eat slowly. Chew, chew, chew. Dump the sugar! Our ancestors certainly did not have sugar (they did not have diabetes or heart disease either!). Eat fish, eat meat, eat chicken, and eat shellfish. By the abundance.

Have a healthy relationship with your body. You are accountable to your body. Make your body the ultimate. Do what's in your power to fix it. If you don't look after your body, where will you live?

Forget the Willpower

Willpower won't help you much when it comes to eating. Get rid of the junk in your fridge and cupboards. Organize your space to keep the crap out and the healthy stuff in. Structure your life so it's easy to eat healthy and hard to eat poorly. You think your willpower will keep you from ripping open that bag of chips after a tough day at work? Make sure the chips aren't there, make sure some crunchy wholemeal crackers are there, and then you won't have that temptation. Be a role model for your loved ones.

Use systems like regular shopping times and meal prep times, and then your food is available when you need it or want it. Figure out dinner around breakfast or lunch time so you don't arrive home ready to snort frozen pizza! If you already have a healthy meal prepared, the decision is made for you and your self-control can return.

Nutritional ketosis is a state of health in which your body is efficiently burning fat as its primary fuel source instead of glucose. When undergoing a ketogenic diet, you are essentially converting yourself from a sugar burner to a fat burner. This is accomplished by reducing your consumption of carbohydrates, increasing your intake of fat, and consuming only an adequate amount of protein to meet your body's needs.

"But don't we need carbs?" you ask. There are essential fatty acids and essential proteins, but there is no such thing as an essential carbohydrate. When the body is in ketosis, it has a glucose sparing effect. First, the muscles burn fatty acids from stored fat in the liver and muscle which spares glucose for the brain to use. Second, once a person is keto-adapted, the brain switches to using ketone bodies for over half of the fuel it needs; as a result, less glucose is necessary since ketone bodies are being used as an alternative fuel. Ketones have been found to have many therapeutic effects on neurons and are being researched intensely in their role for Parkinson's, epilepsy, Alzheimer's, depression, anxiety, and other neurological disorders. Hence, carbohydrates are not essential nutrients.

A ketogenic diet plan requires tracking the carb amounts in the foods you eat and reducing carbohydrate intake to about 20 to 40 grams per day. The nutritional intake on a ketogenic diet typically works out to about 70 to 75 percent of calories from fat, 20 to 25 percent from protein, and 5 to 10 percent from carbohydrate on a daily basis when calories are not restricted.

Filling your plate with green vegetables (spinach, kale, broccoli, and beans), meat, fish, eggs, dairy products low in sugar, and healthy nuts and oils is an essential part of healthy eating. Eating the right quantities of different foods is also important for your overall health.

To correctly implement a ketogenic diet plan is to remember that you are exchanging carbohydrate-containing foods like bread, pasta, and rice with foods with higher fat intake like meats, poultry, fish, avocados, salmon, eggs, bacon, butter, full-fat cream, coconut oil, kidneys, onions, and liver. You need to ensure you have some carbohydrate at each meal but mainly green leafy vegetables.

The amount of meat, chicken, or fish that fits into the palm of your hand is an excellent guide. Try and eat fish at least twice a week. Choose 2–3 servings of milk and milk products each day. These are an excellent source of protein and calcium.

Choose 1–2 cups of green leafy vegetables daily. It's important to stay hydrated as your carbohydrate intake is lowered, since your kidneys will start dumping excess water being retained as a result of the former higher carb intake. Make sure to drink enough water to replace what gets lost. The old 6–8 glasses is a good rule. If you find yourself getting headaches and muscle cramps, you need more water and more minerals such as salt, potassium, and magnesium — the water loss also takes minerals with it. Low carb diet side effects are manageable if you understand why they happen and how to minimize them.

Understanding the reactions will help you avoid the worst of the symptoms. After a few weeks, these side effects will subside as you become keto-adapted and are able to burn fat instead of glucose for fuel.

Here are the most common low carb diet side effects and some tips on how to handle them. After day one or two, you will notice that you are in the bathroom urinating more often. Your body is now burning the extra glycogen (stored glucose) in your liver and muscles. This process releases a lot of water. As mentioned, your kidneys will start eliminating this excess water as your carbohydrate intake and glycogen stores drop. Having lower levels of these minerals may make you drained, dizzy, or lightheaded. You may get muscle cramps and headaches, and you may experience skin itchiness. You should counteract these mineral losses by drinking salty broth, eating foods with potassium (dairy, avocados, and green leafy vegetables), and eating more salt. You should also be sure that your carb intake is below 60 carbs a day and that you have at least 5 grams of salt a day (which is about the same as the standard diet provides). However, if you take medicine for high blood pressure, check with your doctor.

Your weekly shopping list should include some of these foods:

- Two dozen free range eggs (plus more for snacks)
- Two pounds of meat for slow-cooking (beef, pork, or lamb)
- Half a pound of chicken (thighs, skinless, boneless)
- Pink Himalayan rock salt
- Pepper (black or cayenne)
- Two filets of fresh, wild salmon or trout
- One or two 3-ounce packages of smoked salmon
- Ghee
- Two pork chops
- Extra virgin olive oil
- One packet of shrimp
- Extra virgin coconut oil
- Two bunches of asparagus
- Four avocados
- One can of coconut milk

- One jar of green or black olives
- One head of garlic
- One or two jars of sauerkraut
- One package of green beans
- One tin of tuna or salmon
- Lettuce (crunchy types like iceberg)
- Greens of choice (kale, broccoli, spinach, rocket, broccoli
- Sweet potatoes or beetroots
- One package of mushrooms (Portobello or other)
- Bones to make home-made bone broth
- Two medium-sized onions (red or white)
- Celery stalks
- One package of spinach, fresh or frozen
- Coconut or almond milk instead of cream in coffee
- One small bunch of spring onions
- Three packages of cherry tomatoes
- Pastured bacon
- Two 5-ounce packages of blackberries or other berries (fresh or frozen)
- Three or four lemons and limes
- Non-starchy vegetables (cucumber, green pepper, etc.)
- Fresh spices and dried herbs of choice (chives, basil, parsley, rosemary, etc.)
- Oils and fats
- Nuts and seeds (pecans, almonds, walnuts, hazelnuts, macadamias, etc.)
- Vegetables and fruit
- Fermented foods like yogurt, pickles, and kimchi
- Other healthy options like avocado oil, macadamia oil, and olive oil

Summary

It's our ancestral way of eating real, whole, delicious, and nutritious food that encourages weight loss, boosts energy levels, and reduces the risk of diabetes, heart disease, cancer, and chronic illness.

Nutritional ketosis is a state of health in which your body is efficiently burning fat as its primary fuel source instead of glucose. This is accomplished by reducing your consumption of carbohydrates and increasing your intake of fat.

A ketogenic diet plan requires tracking the carbohydrate amounts in the foods eaten and reducing carbohydrate intake to about 20–40 grams per day. The nutritional intake on a ketogenic diet typically works out to about 70–75 percent of calories from fat, 20–25 percent from protein, and 5–10 percent from carbohydrate on a daily basis when calories are not restricted.

Filling your plate with the right quantities of green vegetables (spinach, kale, broccoli, and beans), meat, fish, eggs, dairy products low in sugar, and healthy nuts and oils is an essential part of healthy eating.

That's the ketogenic diet. Once your body has adapted to it, you can look at intermittent fasting to increase weight loss.

Chapter 4

Intermittent Fasting — Timing Your Meals

Once you have become ketone adapted and are reaping the benefits of nutritional ketosis, I believe intermittent fasting is one of the most powerful interventions out there if you're struggling with weight and related health issues. Not only that, but it has been proven to have a beneficial impact on your health and longevity.

Intermittent fasting is becoming very popular because it can help you lose weight without feeling hunger and it contributes to reducing your risk of diseases like heart disease and diabetes. When done correctly, intermittent fasting can also lead to lots of energy and better sleep. Research supports the notion that ditching the "three square meals a day" approach for intermittent fasting may do wonders for your health.

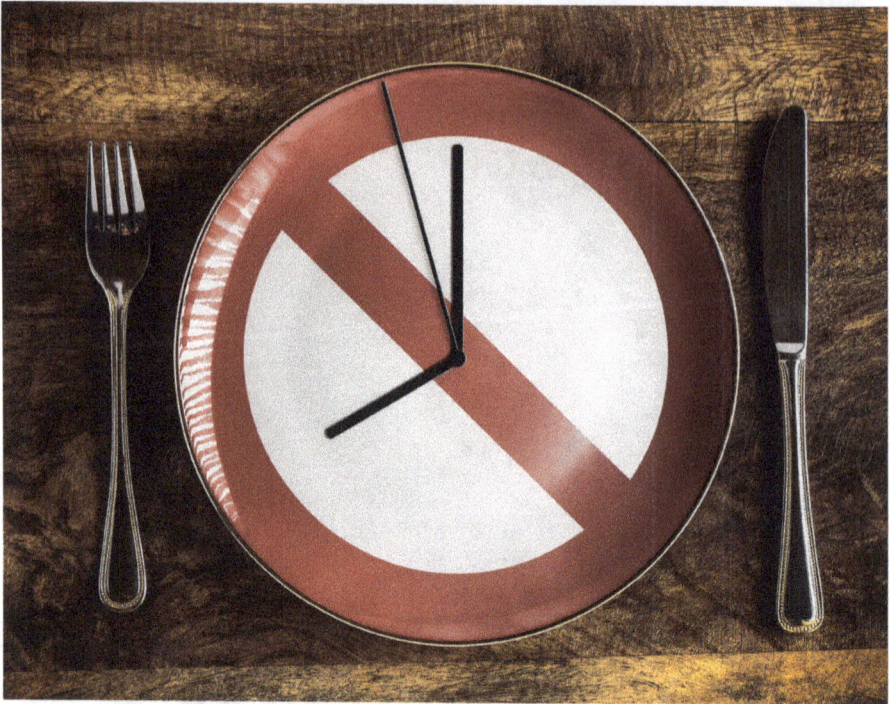

So, what is intermittent fasting exactly? And what are the benefits? To put it simply, intermittent fasting is an eating plan where you adjust your average daily eating times without cutting calories. This helps to:

- Promote insulin sensitivity
- Normalize ghrelin levels, also known as your "hunger hormone"
- Increase the rate of human growth hormone (HGH) production, which has a significant role in health, fitness, and slowing the aging process
- Lower triglyceride levels
- Suppress inflammation and fight free radical damage

Another huge advantage is that exercising in a fasted state can boost fat-burning and help counteract muscle aging and wasting.

The fasting period can range from 13 to 18 hours, because it takes up to six or eight hours for your body to metabolize your glycogen stores. After that, you start to shift to burning fat (a win-win). However, if you are eating every eight hours (or more), you make it far harder for your body to use your fat stores as fuel. During the "fasting state," if your body doesn't have a recently consumed meal to use as energy, it's more likely to pull from the fat stored in your body, rather than the glucose in your blood stream or glycogen in your liver or muscle.

The same goes for working out in a "fasted" state. Without a ready supply of glucose and glycogen to pull from (which has been depleted over the course of your fasted state and hasn't yet been replenished with a pre-workout meal), your body is forced to adapt and pull from the only source of energy available to it — the fat stored in your cells! And the longest you'll ever fast from food is 36 hours.

My personal method is to delay eating for 18 hours after my last meal at night. I would advise that you skip breakfast, eat your lunch and dinner within a six to eight-hour time frame, and stop eating three hours before you go to bed. For example, this means eating only between the hours of 1 pm until 7 pm; just avoid breakfast and make lunch your first meal of the day. You can restrict it even further — down to six, four, or even two hours if you want — but you can still reap many of these rewards by limiting your eating to a six to eight-hour window each day.

Fasting will help your body adjust from burning carbs to burning fat. Eating in a six to eight-hour window can take a few weeks and should be done gradually. Once your body has successfully shifted into fat-burning mode, it will be easier for you to fast for as long as 18 hours and still feel full. Your craving for sugar will slowly dissipate, and you will find it easier to manage your weight.

Within the six to eight hours that you do eat, eliminate refined carbo-hydrates like pizza, bread, and potatoes. Instead, fill your diet with veg-etable carbohydrates, healthy protein, and healthy fats such as butter, eggs, avocado, coconut oil, olive oil, and raw nuts.

While you are restricted to the amount of food you eat during this daily eating plan, I would advise against other versions of intermittent fasting that allow you unlimited junk food when not fasting because it is coun-terproductive. By overindulging on non-fasting days, the health benefits of fasting can easily be lost. What's the point? Intermittent fasting is a lifestyle, not a diet. And it's a lifestyle that includes making healthy food choices whenever you do eat. Also, proper nutrition becomes even more important when fasting, so you want to ensure you have good food choices before you try fasting.

On the days that you work out while fasting, it's best to consume a recovery meal — ideally consisting of the fast-assimilating protein (for example, a three egg omelet fried in olive oil; or three eggs and one avo-cado with sour cream and Himalayan salt; or an almond milk protein shake with a teaspoon of coconut oil whizzed up). I find supplementing magnesium and omega-3 with this meal helps with recovery. Coconut water is a great electrolyte replacement, so you can add that to any meal or shake 30 minutes after your workout.

Finding out what schedule works for you may take some trial and error. It generally takes a month or so to shift to fat burning mode; once you do, your cravings for carbohydrates and unhealthy foods will automati-cally disappear. This is because you're now actually able to burn your stored fat and don't have to rely on new fast-burning carbs for fuel, and ketones is much cleaner energy for the body and the brain than glu-cose. Unfortunately, despite all the evidence, many professionals are still reluctant to prescribe fasting.

Aside from removing your cravings for sugar and snack foods and turning you into an efficient fat-burning machine — thereby making it far easier to maintain a healthy body weight — modern science has confirmed that there are many other good reasons to fast intermittently. For example, research presented at the 2011 Annual Scientific Sessions of the American College of Cardiology in New Orleans showed that fasting triggered a 1,300 percent rise in human growth hormone (HGH) in women and an astounding 2,000 percent in men.

HGH, commonly referred to as "the fitness hormone," plays a significant role in maintaining health, fitness, and longevity, including promotion of muscle growth and boosting fat loss by revving up your metabolism. The fact that it helps build muscle while simultaneously promoting fat loss explains why HGH helps you lose weight without sacrificing muscle mass, and why even athletes can benefit from the practice (as long as they don't overtrain and are careful about their nutrition).

Other health benefits of intermittent fasting include normalizing your insulin and leptin sensitivity (which is crucial for optimal health), normalizing ghrelin levels (also known as "the hunger hormone"), lowering triglyceride levels, reducing inflammation, and lessening free radical damage.

How Intermittent Fasting Has Enormous Benefits for Your Brain

Your brain can also benefit from intermittent fasting. If you don't eat for 10 to 16 hours, your body will go to its fat stores for energy, and fatty acids called ketones will be released into the bloodstream. This has been shown to protect memory and learning ability, as well as slow disease processes in the brain.

Besides releasing ketones as a by-product of burning fat, intermittent fasting also affects brain function by boosting production of a protein called brain-derived neurotrophic factor (BDNF). Research suggests that fasting every other day (restricting your meal on fasting days to about 600 calories), tends to boost BDNF by anywhere from 50 to 400 percent, depending on the brain region. BDNF activates brain stem cells to convert into new neurons, and it triggers numerous other chemicals that promote neural health.

This protein also protects your brain cells from changes associated with Alzheimer's and Parkinson's disease. BDNF also expresses itself in the neuromuscular system where it protects neuromotors from degradation. (The neuromotor is the most critical element in your muscle. Without the neuromotor, your muscle is like an engine without ignition. Neuromotor degradation is part of the process that explains age-related muscle atrophy.)

So, BDNF is actively involved in both your muscles and your brain. This cross-connection appears to be a significant part of the explanation for why a physical workout can have such a beneficial impact on your brain tissue and why the combination of intermittent fasting with high-intensity exercise is a particularly potent combination.

Give Intermittent Fasting a Try

If you're ready to give intermittent fasting a try, consider skipping breakfast, make sure you stop eating and drinking anything but water three hours before you go to sleep, and restrict your eating to a 6 to 8-hour (or less) time frame every day. In the 6-8 hours that you do eat, have healthy protein, minimize your carbs like pasta, bread, and potatoes, and exchange them for healthful fats like butter, eggs, avocado, coconut oil, olive oil, and nuts. This will help shift you from carb-burning mode to fat-burning mode.

Once your body has made this change, it is nothing short of magical as your cravings for sweets and junk food rapidly normalize — if not disappear entirely. Remember, it takes a few weeks, and you have to do it gradually; but once you succeed and switch to fat burning mode, you'll easily be able to fast for 18 hours and not feel hungry. The hunger most people feel is cravings for sugar, and these will disappear once you shift to burning fat instead.

Another side effect and benefit of intermittent fasting is that you will radically improve the beneficial bacteria in your gut. Supporting healthy gut bacteria is one of the most important things you can do to improve your immune system, and it will help you from getting colds or the flu. You will also sleep better, have more energy, have increased mental clarity, and concentrate better. Virtually every aspect of your health will improve as your gut flora becomes balanced.

Based on my experience with intermittent fasting, I believe it's one of the most powerful ways to shift your body into fat burning mode. The effects can be further magnified by exercising while in a fasted state. I have found very few negative side effects with intermittent fasting. The biggest issue I've found, and the biggest concern most people have, is that intermittent fasting will lead to lower energy, lower focus, and the feeling of starvation when you first start. People are concerned they will feel miserable and lethargic and will be ineffective at whatever task they are doing if they don't eat food, especially breakfast — the meal that we have been brainwashed into believing is the most important meal of the day.

However, your body will quickly adapt to intermittent fasting. While the initial transition is a bit of a jolt, you will soon find you have more energy and will function just as well eating only a couple of times a day.

Summary

When taking up intermittent fasting, start by fasting from morning until noon, and then add an hour or two per day. In a matter of weeks, you will be used to this way of eating and be feeling great.

Practice this twice a week, increasing to three or four days a week, and then five or six days once you are fully adapted.

Take your time with the adaption period; some people can jump straight in while others need more time. You will experience amazing results quite quickly, both physically and mentally.

That's it for intermittent fasting, but we haven't finished with food. Next, we will look at the addictions created by food.

Chapter 5

Food Addiction

A Medical Condition

I believe food addiction should be recognized as a medical condition so overweight people can get help to quit. Research shows that over a third of us could be addicted to food. And yet, struggling addicts received no funding or support, whereas people at the other end of the spectrum receive help for eating disorders like anorexia.

Food addiction is very similar to several other eating disorders, including binge eating disorder and bulimia. When the world discovers that refined sugar is just another white powder, along with pure cocaine, it will change our minds and attitude towards refined foods.

Much like drug addicts, people addicted to junk food need increasingly significant "hits" to get their daily fix. Even though they know it's not right, they still just feel this drive to eat. More than one-third (35.7 percent) of adults are obese. More than 1 in 20 (6.3 percent) have extreme obesity. Almost 3 in 4 men (74 percent) are overweight or obese. The prevalence of obesity is similar for both men and women (about 36 percent).

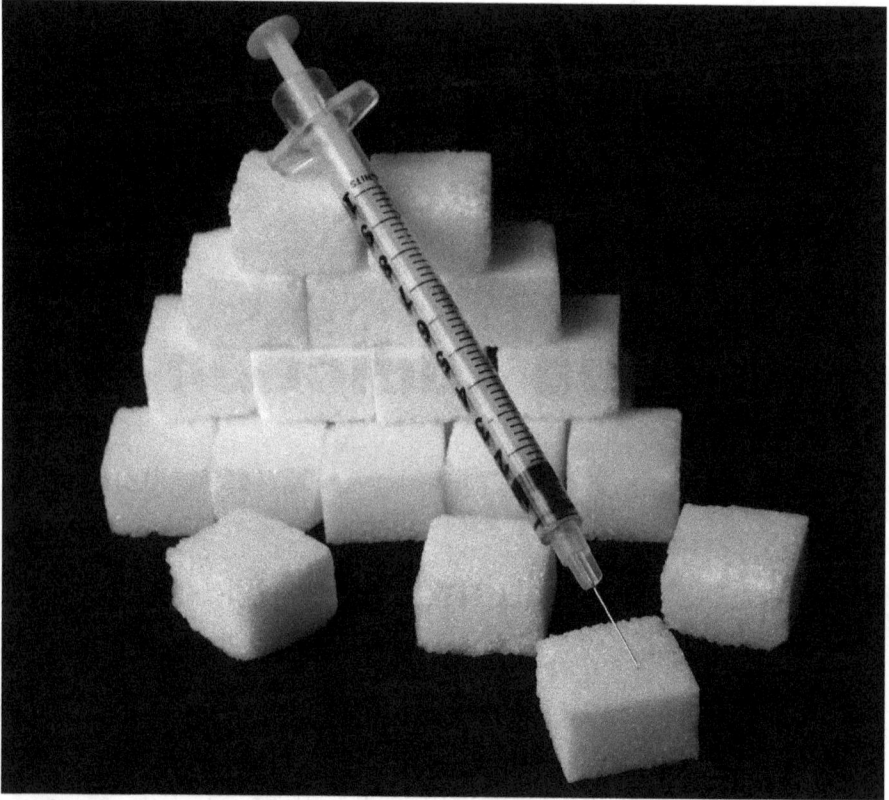

It seems we are in the midst of an advancing obesity epidemic. There are no medical or blood tests available to diagnose food addiction; it is based on behavioral symptoms, just like other addictions. A former smoker who has one puff of a cigarette will more likely become addicted again — instantly. An alcoholic who has one glass of wine will more likely relapse, with all the dreadful consequences that follow. There is no way of getting around it. This is how addiction works. The only thing that reliably works against addiction is complete abstinence. Obviously, with food abstinence isn't the answer, but control is. The sooner you accept that, the sooner you will recover.

It seems impossible to avoid the wrong foods completely. These foods are a major part of our culture and are everywhere, but once you've made the decision to never eat them again, avoiding them becomes easier. You can prepare yourself and make the transition as easy as possible by doing the following.

Trigger foods

Write down a list of the unhealthy foods you tend to binge on or crave. These are the trigger foods you need to avoid altogether.

Fast food

Write down a list of food places that serve healthy food. It's imperative and will prevent relapse when you find yourself hungry and not in the mood to cook.

Don't worry

It's important not to worry about weight gain. Conquering your addiction is hard enough. By adding extra restrictions and hunger to the cocktail, you will definitely make things even harder and set yourself up for failure. Allow two to three months for this transitional time.

Set a date and stick with it

Set a date — sooner rather than later. (Monday always works for me.) From this day onward, promise yourself that you will never touch the addictive foods again. Not a single bite. Ever. Period.

Get help if you need it

When all else fails, seek help. Most people have had a failed attempt before they succeed in the long term. But if you find that you are relapsing often, it could be a sign that you need help. Luckily, help is not far off. There are support groups and health professionals that can help you overcome this serious problem.

There are several free options available as well — including 12 step programs like Overeaters Anonymous, Food Addicts Anonymous (FAA), and Food Addicts in Recovery Anonymous (FA). Go to their websites, find a meeting (they also have online Skype sessions), and go to it. Another avenue is to search for treatment options in your area. Get on the internet and search for something like food addiction treatment + the name of your city. The chances are good that you will find something that suits you. Whatever you do, do something!

Summary

If you think you fit the description of a food addict — seek help. Life will improve and be more enjoyable. Food addiction should be recognized as a medical condition so overweight people can get help to quit. Write down a list of food places that serve healthy food. It's imperative and will prevent relapse when you find yourself hungry and not in the mood to cook.

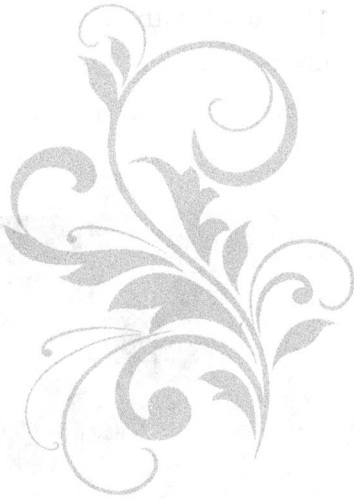

Chapter 6

Creating the Right Mindset

The Power of the Mind

If you think you can, you will. If you think you will fail, you will. Your mind is incredibly powerful. I believe you are what you think. The power of positive thinking is fundamental to your success. I have seen the results when we use the power of our mind backed by education and information.

Let's look at the mind. The law of attraction simply states that "like attracts like." Following the law of attraction, you attract into your life the things, circumstances, and conditions that correspond to the nature of your habitual thoughts and beliefs, both conscious and subconscious.

Every area of your life, including your weight, health, relationships, and finances are influenced by this great universal law that "like attracts like." This means you are likely getting whatever your subconscious mind is focusing on.

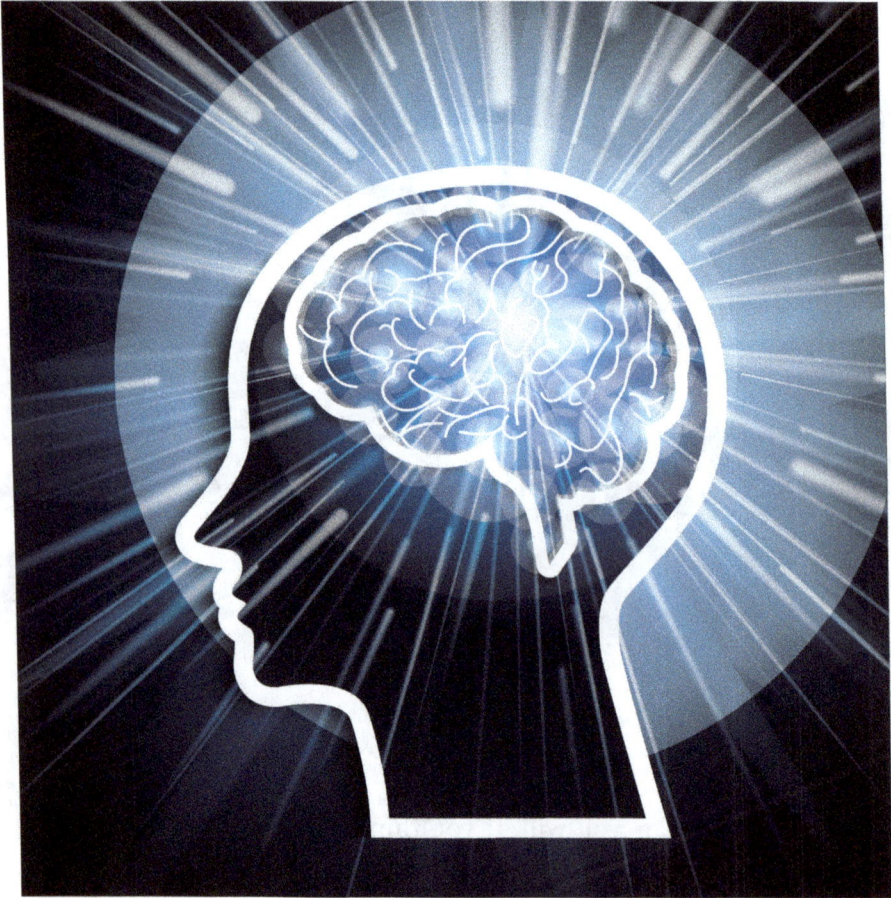

A positive attitude attracts positive experiences and circumstances, while a negative attitude attracts those conditions that we deem harmful or unwanted. By visualizing a mental image of what you want to achieve, or by repeating positive affirmations, you create and bring into your life what you visualize or repeat in your mind. In other words, you use the power of your mind, thoughts, imagination, and words to influence your world.

Researchers analyzed data from a study of patients who had their arms in casts. During the study, half of the patients imagined exercise with their broken arm and the other half didn't. When the casts were removed, those who had imagined exercising had twice as much strength in that arm as those who hadn't.

Yes, the imagining of motion, which occurs in the same part of the brain where the impulse to move originates, does have physical benefits. And, while it's not a substitute for real exercise, imaginary exercise has been shown to improve the performance of those who do highly physical jobs — like surgeons, athletes, and musicians.

Take one day at a time. Small steps. Just because you put the law of attraction in place and start shifting your thoughts and beliefs does not magically mean that you will become thin and toned. There is still the action and effort of doing. You still need to do the work yourself, but visualization motivates you towards your goals.

In the end, your goals will come down to *just doing it* one day at a time. Each day you have to keep telling yourself who you are. Write down your goals and read them before you get out of bed in the morning. Surround yourself with images that create positive emotion. Find that one picture that personally represents feeling great and looking great. Put that picture where you can see it. Make sure there are strong emotions attached to it, so it is branded in your subconscious. Visualize yourself often with your new look, and say to yourself as often as you can in the mirror, "I love my newly transformed body." These affirmations are very powerful, and there is no doubt that there will be a positive shift in your energy levels and attitude, making you feel great.

Don't underestimate emotional support, either. Whether it's a personal trainer, a close friend, a work colleague, or a support group, surround yourself with people who are working towards the same goal. If you can't find a group, then create a group yourself. Take positive action towards your goals. This is the best way to defeat an adverse environment. You will have to avoid negative talk like "I can't" or "I have failed before," because you can do it. You must choose to think positive. Remember that these new dialogues in your head will have no meaning if they are not backed up with action.

What is the one thing you have that can change your life today? *Choice.* Everybody has a choice, and choice = destiny. Quitters never win, and winners never quit! Bottom line: you need to start living and breathing the lifestyle that will take you to your goals.

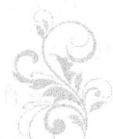

Summary

If you believe you can, you will. If you believe you can't, you won't! Change your thought pattern.

The law of attraction is very powerful. You attract into your life circumstances and conditions that correspond to the nature of your habitual thoughts and beliefs, both conscious and subconscious.

By visualizing a mental image of what you want to achieve, or by repeating positive affirmations, you can create and bring those positives into your life. Each day you must keep telling yourself who you are. Write down your goals and read them before you get out of bed in the morning. Surround yourself with images that create positive emotion.

As Nike says "Just Do It."

Chapter 7

Diabetes

One of the World's Biggest Killers

The world is facing a perpetual march of diabetes that now affects nearly one in 11 adults, according to the World Health Organization. As the world's waistlines have ballooned — with one in three people now overweight — so too has the number of diabetes cases. Failing to control levels of sugar in the blood has devastating health consequences. It triples the risk of a heart attack and leaves people 20 times more likely to have a leg amputated, as well as increases the risk of stroke, kidney failure, blindness, and complications in pregnancy.

Diabetes itself is the eighth biggest killer in the world. It accounts for 1.5 million deaths annually, with a further 2.2 million deaths linked to high blood sugar levels. 43 percent of the deaths were before the age of 70.

In the 1980s, the highest rates of diabetes were found in affluent countries. But, in a remarkable transformation, it is now low and middle-income countries bearing the largest burden. That's where we see the steepest increase. Knowing that's where most of the population lives in the world, this shows that the numbers will continue to grow unless drastic action is taken.

It is only by keeping blood sugar levels in check that the life-threatening complications of the disease can be contained.

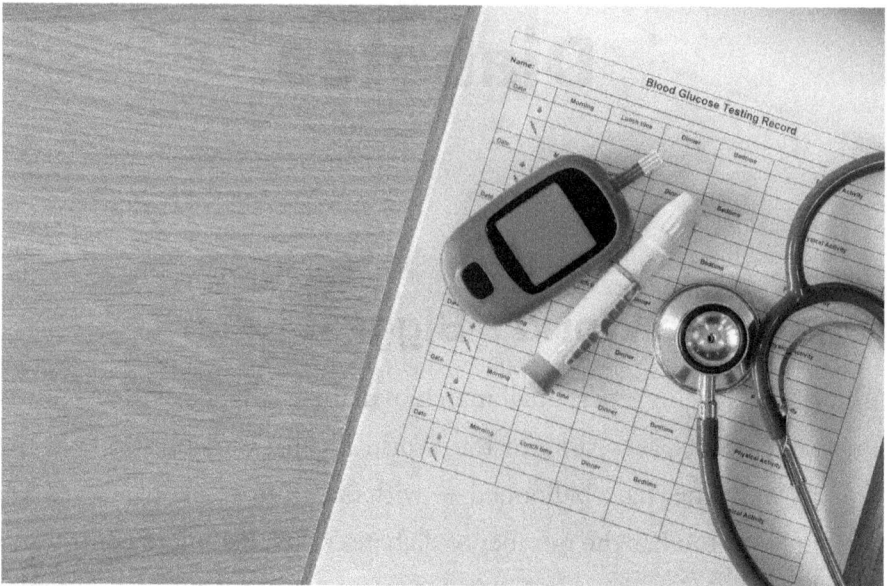

The Signs and Symptoms

The International Diabetes Foundation highlights common signs and symptoms that should prompt someone to get tested for diabetes as soon as possible:

Excessive thirst and frequent urination

Have you been going to the bathroom to urinate more often recently? Do you notice that you spend most of the day going to the toilet?

When there is too much glucose (sugar) in your blood, you will urinate more often. If your insulin is ineffective, or not there at all, your kidneys cannot filter the glucose back into the blood. The kidneys will take water from your blood to dilute the glucose, which in turn fills up your bladder. If you are urinating more than usual, you will need to replace that lost liquid. You will be drinking more than usual.

Intense hunger

Since the insulin in your blood is not working properly (or is not there at all) and your cells are not getting their energy, your body may react by trying to find more energy — food. Because of this, you will become hungry.

Blurred vision

Blurred vision can be caused by tissue being pulled from your eye lenses. This affects your eyes' ability to focus. This can be treated, but there are severe cases where blindness or prolonged vision problems can occur.

Diagnosis and Treatment

Diabetes is diagnosed by blood tests, which can be organized through your doctor. If you are very unwell, you should seek medical assistance immediately. Your doctor will advise you on what treatment is best for you, but whatever this may be, healthy food choices and staying active are important.

The goal is to lower your blood glucose and improve your body's use of insulin. This is achieved through healthy diet and exercise, which helps people with diabetes get off a blood sugar roller coaster. The roller coaster happens when blood sugars rise to absurdly high levels after a high carb meal and then crash to low levels when large amounts of insulin are secreted or injected. A ketogenic diet treats diabetes at the cause and is a much safer, more efficient plan than injecting insulin to counteract the consumption of high carb foods. Implementing the ketogenic is worth it, as explained earlier in Chapter 3.

You may also want to take 400 mg of magnesium citrate every night before bed. (Check with your doctor first if you have kidney or heart health issues.) The intake of magnesium has shown to reduced the risk for blood sugar and metabolic problems by a massive 71%. Higher magnesium intake reduces the risk of insulin metabolism and impaired glucose. It slows the progression from pre-diabetes to diabetes in middle - aged Americans. If you are at a high risk of diabetes magnesium intake will be highly beneficial. People with insulin resistance also experience more excretion of magnesium in their urine, which further diminishes magnesium levels. An estimated 80% of Americans are magnesium deficient. It's also really important to eat at least two cups of green leafy vegetables every day. These vegetables not only provide magnesium but potassium and vitamin K, which will also help with hunger.

As your body goes through the process of reprogramming itself to burn fat instead of sugar, there's a transition period of about 2–21 days where carb cravings will be worse. These will subside and eventually disappear — as long as you don't cheat. Eating a lot of carbs will bring the cravings right back. And for most of us, eating sugar in any amount will start the slide down the slippery slope to carb overload.

I put together the following list of tips on how to stop sugar cravings for those people with diabetes to get off the blood sugar roller coaster. I know how powerful these urges can be, and it's tough to fight them when they are raging away at your brain. These tips are useful when first starting a ketogenic, low carb diet, and they can help you get past the rough spots on your way to a better diet and to feeling great.

Stop Sugar Cravings

Sugar cravings, like most addictions, are frequently the result of unbalanced blood and brain chemistry, and these tips help because they work toward correcting such imbalances.

Tip #1

Make a quick tuna salad with canned tuna and some full-fat mayonnaise. Tuna is a great food choice for your diabetes diet, providing you with omega 3 fatty acids, protein, vitamin D, and other important nutrients. This will not spike your blood sugar levels because it contains no carbohydrates. Mayonnaise is satiating and delicious. Together this is a sugar craving crusher.

Tip #2

If you have sugar cravings and want to satisfy your sweet tooth safely, Stevia is your best bet. It's a natural sweetener that has zero calories, is 300 times sweeter than sugar, and doesn't raise blood sugar levels. Add it to some plain Greek yogurt or your coffee.

Tip #3

Daily exercise increases the amount of a neurotransmitter called dopamine in your brain. Higher levels of dopamine are associated with better moods and reduced sugar cravings. Get up off the couch and go for a walk. Simply moving more and sitting less can boost your health. All those little movements add up.

Sitting for extended periods of time has been linked with heart disease, diabetes, cancer, and obesity. Getting up hourly and walking to the bathroom, getting a refill of water, or standing up to stretch can decrease stiffness, boost energy, and burn calories. When watching TV, get up and move during commercial breaks. Do a few stretches, walk around the house. When going about your day, take the stairs instead of elevators and escalators.

Recent research published in the Archives of Internal Medicine found that non-exercise activity thermogenesis (NEAT) is the kind of energy used walking to work, typing, gardening, fidgeting, and undertaking other non-formal exercise tasks.

Adopting (NEAT) behaviors can increase daily caloric expenditure by as much as 350 calories per day and is particularly beneficial for obese individuals.

Tip #4

Consuming fermented foods is one of the most effective and healthiest ways to reduce or eliminate sugar cravings. Our modern diets are devoid of the sour taste, and bringing it back into the diet can help to regulate appetite. More importantly, the microflora (the good bacteria and yeast, also called probiotics) in fermented foods and drinks help balance the inner ecosystem and reduce or eliminate cravings.

Tip #5

Take supplements to help your body control blood sugar. Supplements like B vitamin complex, biotin, alpha lipoic acid, zinc, vitamin E, and chromium GTF are all helpful in controlling blood sugar fluctuations.

Summary

Keeping blood sugar levels in check means the life-threatening complications of diabetes can be contained. Whether you have diabetes or want to prevent it, a ketogenic diet treats diabetes at the cause and can be a much safer and efficient plan than injecting insulin to counteract the consumption of high carbohydrate foods.

It's also really important to stop sugar cravings in their tracks by eating right and exercising every day. Eat at least two cups of raw green leafy vegetables daily and keep moving. Take the stairs instead of the elevator or park farther away from the store to fit a short walk into your schedule. Simply moving more and sitting less can improve your health.

Chapter 8

The Brain

Could careful attention to diet and exercise help protect the aging brain from problems with nerve cell signals involved in memory and cognition? Sorry, but as you get into this section, you might come across some large words (unless you are an expert). They are necessary to explain the process.

Developments in this area of the aging brain could significantly affect the millions of baby boomers who are now facing retirement. Their quality of life, independence, and even economic status will largely be defined by their ability to process information as they age.

In researching the nutrition-brain connection, new technologies are being developed and used to do things like take images of the brain or count individual brain cells. Behavioral tests that measure motor and cognitive skills — or lack thereof — are also providing valuable insights. The science of nutrition and brain function is relatively new and evolving.

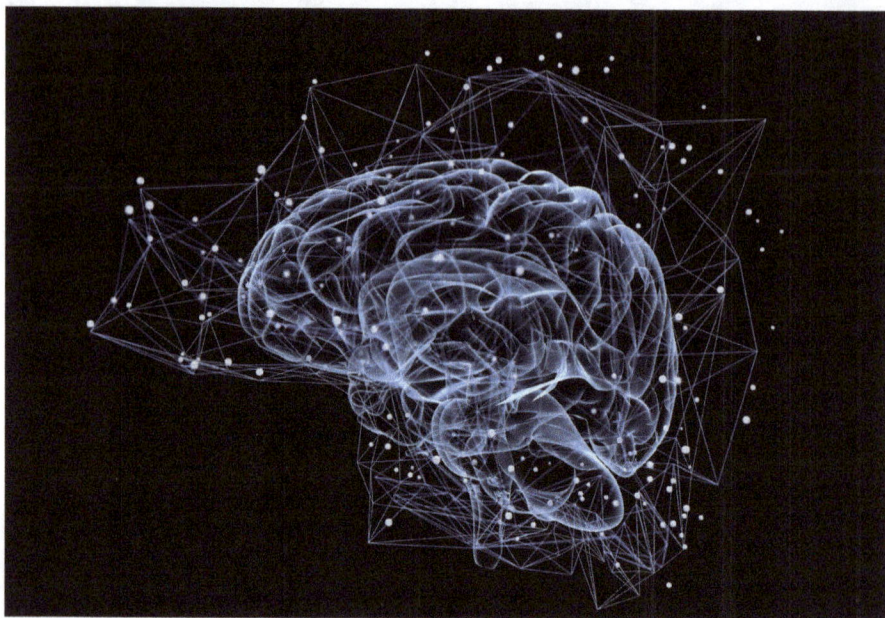

Nutrition for the Mind

Before dealing with improved nutrition for the mind, we need to understand a little about how the brain works. In short, the brain is a network of neurons, which are specialized nerve cells with branches that connect to thousands of other neurons. Scientists call this dense branching network a "neuron forest."

To get an idea of just how complex this is, let's look at the Amazon rainforest. The Amazon covers 2 million square miles and contains 100 billion trees with more than 100 trillion leaves. The rather surprising news is that there are as many cells in our brain as there are trees in the Amazon and as many connections as leaves.

The connections between each neuron are called dendrites. Where one neuron meets another, there is a gap, much like a spark plug, called a synapse. It is within the synapse that messages are sent from one neuron to the other. The words the brain uses to send messages from one cell to another are called neurotransmitters, and the letters are built from amino acids.

We have around 60,000 thoughts a day — most of them repeats! With every thought, we have, there is a ripple of activity across the network of nerves called your brain. The message is sent from one sending station and received in a receiving station called a receptor.

The brain needs a constant supply of protein and energy to maintain all this activity. Any imbalance in the uptake of protein or energy to the brain and you can experience fatigue, mood swings, irritability, crying spells, poor concentration, forgetfulness, dizziness, excessive thirst, and blurred vision. This energy comes from ketones being broken down from fats [ketogenic diet] or proteins being broken down into amino acids.

Ketogenic diets, which are low in carbohydrates and high in protein and essential fat, have been prescribed for seizures for a long time. Protein is vital since all neurotransmitters are made directly from it. The quality of protein is determined by its balance of amino acids. You can change your mood by the protein you eat. Here are the amino acids.

Amino Acids:
The Alphabet for Mind and Mood

Protein is converted by the body into amino acids. They improve the brain's "talking mechanism." There are nine essential amino acids that then convert into the 23 amino acids needed for optimum brain function. These are:

- Threonine
- Tryptophan
- Methionine
- Valine
- Phenylalanine
- Isoleucine
- Lysine
- Leucine
- Histidine

These amino acids are converted by the body into neurotransmitters. For example, the neurotransmitters dopamine, noradrenaline, and adrenaline are made from the amino acid phenylalanine. These are your motivational and feel good neurotransmitters, so eating foods like eggs and fish will improve your up and go.

The neurotransmitter GABA is made from taurine. GABA is your calming neurotransmitter. GABA is the metabolic byproduct of plants and microorganisms. While GABA is not found in fresh food, it can be found in certain fermented foods, and these foods can stimulate your body to produce more of it. Fermented cabbage and sauerkraut are great for this.

The neurotransmitter serotonin is made from the amino acid tryptophan. Serotonin is known to help improve your mood, so eating foods like eggs and soy protein rich in tryptophan can help your moods.

For the conversion of amino acids to neurotransmitters to be effective, the brain depends on intelligent nutrients to do this. These include vitamins and minerals, which are like the people behind the scene of a great play. Without them, the play would not go on.

So, different amino acids make different neurotransmitters. They deal with the processing of your 60,000 thoughts each day, which means that you will suffer if there are any imbalances. To understand why amino acids are your brain's best friend, we need to delve into what neurotransmitters do.

The Jobs of Neurotransmitters

There are hundreds of various neurotransmitters, but we're only going to discuss the main players in the orchestra of your brain.

Tryptamine, serotonin

Tryptamine and serotonin promote and enhance sleep, improve self-esteem, relieve depression, diminish cravings, and prevent agitated depression and worrying. Foods rich in these are lamb, beef, fish, pork, chicken, dairy, nuts, seeds, and eggs.

Adrenaline, noradrenaline

Adrenaline and noradrenaline promote enthusiasm, excitement, happiness, alertness, and motivation. Not only do they work as antidepressants, but they also help appetite control, energy, and sexual arousal. Foods that help release these are eggs, meat, cottage cheese, turkey, chicken, yogurt, tuna, and seafood. Vegetarian choices include tofu, beans, peas, lentils, and soy products.

Dopamine

Dopamine helps monitor the brain's reward and pleasure centers. Dopamine also helps regulate movement and emotional responses, and it enables us not only to see rewards but to take action to move toward them. Dopamine deficiency can result in Parkinson's disease, and people with low dopamine activity may be more prone to addiction. The presence of a certain kind of dopamine receptor is also associated with sensation-seeking people, more commonly known as "risk takers." Foods that boost dopamine are eggs, kale, and fish.

GABA (Gamma Amino Butyric Acid)

GABA is found throughout the central nervous system and is associated with anti-stress, anti-anxiety, anti-panic, anti-pain, maintaining control, and focus. Foods to boost GABA are broccoli, almonds, spinach, beef liver, and walnuts.

Acetylcholine

Acetylcholine promotes alertness, memory, sexual performance, and appetite control, and it helps in the release of growth hormone. Dairy, chicken, fish, and meat are all foods that can boost acetylcholine.

What we eat affects everything from our production of neurotransmitters and hormones, to our energy levels, and our response to stress and the demands of daily living. There is an important connection between the foods you eat and the neurotransmitters your brain produces.

Foods That Boost Your Brain Power

Phospholipids

Phospholipids are intelligent fats and your memory's best friend. They are the insulation experts. They help improve your mind, mood, and mental performance and protect against age-related memory decline and Alzheimer's. There are three types of phospholipids: phosphatidylcholine, phosphatidylserine, and phosphatidyl dimethylethanolamine.

Phosphatidylcholine

Phosphatidylcholine (PC) is probably the most important phospholipid that supplies the brain with the nutrient choline. Choline is needed to make acetylcholine, a vital neurotransmitter for memory, control of sensory input signals, and muscular control. Acetylcholine is abundant or highly concentrated in the hippocampus.

People with Alzheimer's disease show a marked deficiency of acetylcholine. Even if memory is intact if you don't have enough acetylcholine you can't connect one part of the memory with other regions. For example, you remember the face but can't remember the name. You can grow the hippocampus to prevent memory loss and Alzheimer's. People with large hippocampus do not get Alzheimer's disease — even if they have Alzheimer's in the brain. So, eating foods rich in phosphatidylcholine and supplementing choline has been proven to boost memory.

The recommended dose is 250 mg to 500 mg a day for general health purposes. Doses should be taken to suit the individual, as too high of a dose may give the user a headache. It is suggested that doses start out at 50 to 100 mg a day and that users adjust upwards by their tolerance. Another source of choline is lecithin granules, which can be sprinkled on food. The lecithin should contain more than 30 percent of phosphatidylcholine, so read the label first.

Foods rich in PC are omega-rich eggs, seeds, and fish (especially tuna and sardines).

Phosphatidylserine

Phosphatidylserine (PS) is the memory molecule. Phosphatidylserine is considered to be a principal agent in providing nourishment and support to the brain. Phosphatidylserine provides strength to the memory and can rejuvenate the brain cells membrane of the individual.

Phosphatidylserine is found to boost the learning capabilities of the person, and it also relieves depression. In the human body, phosphatidylserine is of great importance because it increases the number of membrane receptor sites for receiving the chemical messages.

Scientific studies reveal that phosphatidylserine is essential for releasing neurotransmitters. These neurotransmitters are important for the proper communication of the brain with the other parts of the body. Phosphatidylserine also stimulates the brain to produce dopamine. Dopamine plays a critical role in reducing stress and depression. Phosphatidylserine is essential for the efficient neurotransmission. Proper levels of phosphatidylserine in the human body protect the individual from stroke and unconsciousness.

The recommended dose is supplemental phosphatidylserine (**100 mg** three times daily). Foods rich in PS are; chicken heart, herring, tuna, chicken leg with skin, chicken liver, and salmon.

Phosphatidyl dimethylethanolamine

Phosphatidyl dimethylethanolamine (DMAE) is a natural brain stimulant. DMAE reduces anxiety, stops the mind from racing, improves concentration, promotes learning, and acts as a mild brain stimulant. It can also protect neurons and other cells from harmful effects of certain types of oxidation. It does this by embedding itself in the structure of the cell and acting as an antioxidant, as well as sustaining metabolic processes in the body through a process known as methyl donation.

The ideal dose for memory improvement is 100 mg or more, taken in the morning or midday, not in the evening. DMAE can take up to three weeks to work, so immediate results are not evident, but they are worth waiting for. Food sources are fish, particularly anchovies and sardines.

All three of these phospholipids are equally important for the building of receptor stations and receiving stations, but they are not the whole story when it comes to brain food. I hope you are ready for some more unpronounceable names.

Pyroglutamate

This is the master of communication. Pyroglutamic acid is an amino acid that researchers have found highly concentrated in the spinal fluid and human brain that can improve concentration, learning, memory, and the speed of reflexes. The brain-stimulating benefits of pyroglutamic acid have been known for several years.

As early as 1984, Italian researchers reported that pyroglutamic acid encouraged the release of the memory chemical acetylcholine in the brain. Pyroglutamate does three things that help memory and mental alertness.

It increases the production of acetylcholine, it increases the number of receptors for acetylcholine, and it improves communication between the left and right hemispheres of the brain. In other words, pyroglutamate improves the brain's talking, listening, and cooperation.

Pyroglutamate is found in many foods, including fish, dairy products, fruit, and vegetables. The most common form found in supplements is arginine pyroglutamate. Supplement 400 mg to 1000 mg a day for optimal brain function.

Prostaglandins

Prostaglandins are extremely active hormone-like substances. They relax blood vessels, and therefore lower blood pressure. They maintain water balance. They boost immunity. They decrease inflammation and pain and help insulation work. In the brain, they regulate the release of neurotransmitters, and low levels of prostaglandins are known to be involved in various conditions such as schizophrenia, Alzheimer's, and depression.

Essential fats, omega-3 and omega-6, are broken down by the body into prostaglandins. These fats are critical for the brain's function and structure. Low levels have been linked to schizophrenia, depression, and learning problems. Evening Primrose oil has high levels of omega-6. Evening Primrose Oil was given to Alzheimer's patients in a controlled trial, and significant improvement in memory and mental performance were found. These results were made even more spectacular when vitamin C, B1, B3, and zinc were added — all of which are needed to help convert essential fats into prostaglandins. We should have about equal or twice as many omega-6 fats as omega-3 fats. For omega-3, this means taking either concentrated fish oil capsules with eicosapentaenoic acid (EPA) and docosahexaenoic acid (DHA) or flaxseed oil capsules. Krill oil, like fish oil, contains these omega-3 fats; The recommended dose is 1,000 milligrams a day (two 500 mg capsules). This is based, in part, on clinical trials that showed benefits at this dose. And for omega 6 a relatively small amount of oil, amounting to about three grams or four 750 mg capsules of Evening Primrose Oil (EPO), for a 150-pound adult.

Vitamins and minerals

Without these, the body and the brain cannot turn all the essential nutrients into what the body and the brain need. One of their primary roles is to turn glucose into energy, amino acids into neurotransmitters, essential fats into prostaglandins, and choline and serine into phospholipids.

We know that vitamins and minerals improve IQ. How? Adults and children can think faster and concentrate for longer with the optimal uptake of vitamins and minerals. Studies have shown every one of the 50 nutrients plays a significant role in promoting mental health. Here are the main players:

Thiamine (B1)

All of the B vitamins are water soluble, meaning the body does not store them. Vitamin B1 helps turn glucose into energy; one of the first signs of deficiency is tiredness, fatigue, and poor concentration and attention. Food sources of thiamine include liver, beef, nuts, milk, nuts, eggs, pork, legumes, peas, and yeast.

Niacin (B3), pyridoxine (B6), folic acid (B9), and cobalamin (B12)

These four B vitamins are your brain's best friends. They "oil the wheels" of the brain's neurotransmitters, especially dopamine, adrenaline, noradrenaline, and serotonin. The Neurotransmitters are the brain's chemicals of communication, sending messages from one brain cell to another. Without enough of these vital B vitamins, the brain cannot produce chemicals, and that can make you feel crazy. This is because they help control "methylation," a chemical process that goes on throughout the brain and body, contributing to turning one neurotransmitter into another.

First is Niacin or vitamin B3. Of all nutrients connected to mental health, this one is the most famous. The deficiency of B3 was discovered to be the cause of pellagra, a disease in which people developed mental illness, diarrhea, and eczema.

Niacin has been extensively researched in the treatment of acute schizophrenia and has been highly effective in doses of several grams; the recommended daily allowance is 18 mg! Getting enough niacin does more than stop you from developing psychosis. In one study, 141 mg daily improved memory by more than 10 percent in both young and old. Food sources are fish, poultry, organ meats, peanuts, legumes, broccoli, carrots, avocados, tomatoes, and eggs.

Second and third is pyridoxine and folic acid, or vitamin B6 and B9. A lot of us are deficient in B6 and B9. Supplementation showed significant improvement in patients that were both depressed and schizophrenic. B9 deficiency is very common in patients with mental health conditions. Lack of B6 means you won't make serotonin as efficiently, which could potentially lead to depression. B6 can help relieve stress too. To keep your B6 and B9 at optimal levels, try eating more organ meats, eggs, chicken, fish, brewer's yeast, carrots, peas, spinach, sunflower seeds, and walnuts.

Fourth on the list is [cobalamin] B12, which is also vital for a healthy nervous system. Without B12, neither the brain nor the nervous system can work properly. Deficiency has been shown to be present in as many as half the patients with dementia, with an equivalent number indicating an inability to absorb it. However, it's not just the older people who need it. Low levels cause poor mental performance in adolescents too. Food source include protein-bound in animal foods, fish, eggs, dairy products, meats, salmon, tuna, chicken, lamb, beef, milk, and cheese.

Pantothenic Acid (B5)

Vitamin B5 is crucial to the manufacture of red blood cells, as well as stress-related hormones and sex hormones produced in the adrenal glands — small glands that sit atop the kidneys. Vitamin B5 is also important in maintaining a healthy digestive tract, and it helps the body use other vitamins. Vitamin B5 deficiency is rare but may include symptoms such as depression, fatigue, irritability, insomnia, stomach pains, burning feet, and upper respiratory infections.

The best sources of vitamin B5 are kale, brewer's yeast, avocados, cauliflower, tomatoes, broccoli, lentils, beef (especially organ meats such as kidney and liver), egg yolks, turkey, chicken, duck, milk, peanuts, split peas, soybeans, sunflower seeds, sweet potatoes, lobster, wheat germ, and salmon. Vitamin B5 can be found in multivitamins and B-complex vitamins.

Summary

Protein is vital for mental health since all neurotransmitters are made directly from it. The quality of protein is determined by its balance of amino acids. You can change your mood by the protein you eat. Milk, eggs, beef, cheese, yogurt, fish, and chicken are complete proteins — so a diet rich in these foods is a must.

Fish, poultry, organ meats, peanuts, legume, broccoli, carrots, avocados, tomatoes, nuts, pork, and eggs are rich in B vitamins, which are essential for mental health. Essential fats, omega-3 and omega-6, are broken down by the body into prostaglandins. These fats are critical for the brain's function and structure. Low levels have been linked to schizophrenia depression and learning problems.

Supplementing omega-3, and omega-6 significantly improves memory and mental performance. These results were made even more spectacular when vitamin C, B1, B3, and zinc were added — all of which are needed to help convert essential fats into prostaglandins.

Chapter 9

Depression and Hypoglycemia

Depression is a complex problem, but many so-called experts do not recognize and are not aware of the nutritional aspects of depression. I find this most frustrating when it is well known that the precursors to the brain's neurotransmitters, and their enzymes and coenzymes (vitamins and minerals), all derive from the food we eat. We cannot expect psychotherapy to be of much help if depression is a biological disorder.

Prescription drugs do not treat the underlying biochemical imbalance, and most patients are advised that they may have to take drugs for a predetermined period. This is not a positive future with the inevitable side effects of drugs. The brain is an enormous factory of activity. It consumes

40 percent of all energy consumed, and it consumes even more when we are studying or learning. The brain is 60 percent fat, so it's essential that we eat healthy fats to feed our brain.

All components of the brain are constantly being replaced. Some take years, some take months, but one of the most important components, docosahexaenoic acid (an omega-3 fatty acid), is replaced very rapidly — in about two weeks. This means that, if you don't replace the nutrient, your brain can not function properly. A deficiency in omega-3 fatty acids will result in depression, anxiety, chronic fatigue, memory loss, and personality change.

To avoid this, make sure your daily diet includes things like salmon, sardines, eggs, beef, sunflower oil, nuts, avocado, and olive oil.

Natural Remedy

In addition to consuming the required foods, there is a natural remedy for depression that may help treat a wide variety of conditions related to low serotonin levels. Hydroxytryptophan, or 5-HTP, is a chemical that the body makes from tryptophan (an essential amino acid that you get from food). After tryptophan is converted into 5-HTP, the chemical changes into serotonin (a neurotransmitter that relays signals between brain cells).

5-HTP dietary supplements help raise serotonin levels in the brain. Since serotonin helps regulate mood and behavior, 5-HTP may have a positive effect on mood, sleep, appetite, anxiety, and pain sensation. Healthcare professionals recommend 50 mg of 5-HTP taken one to three times per day. Some studies have used higher doses, but because 5-HTP can be toxic at high doses, you should talk to your doctor before raising the dose. Your health care provider can help determine the right treatment for you. For depression or anxiety, the dose can be 150 to 300 mg daily.

Sugar's Role

In the Western world, with the high sugar consumption hidden in all foods, we should not be surprised to find a connection between sugar and depression. Why does sugar cause such an avalanche in the brain?

When the blood sugar is too high, the body releases an excess amount of insulin to remove blood sugar. The person is then hypoglycemic (which means they have low blood sugar). This stimulates adrenaline, noradrenaline, and glutamate, which are your hormones that make you excitable, jittery, and nervous when your blood sugar falls.

This sounds like a long process, but it happens in a blink of an eye. These crazy fluctuations in blood sugar levels, along with stress hormones and insulin levels, are said to be responsible for the mood swings, phobias, anxiety attacks, violence, alcoholism, insomnia, drug addiction, shakes, and all forms of mental illness.

Studies have shown that hypoglycemia (low blood sugar) is common in psychiatric patients and criminals. There is a 74 percent incidence of people with hypoglycemia having anxiety that is associated with schizophrenia. Also, 60 percent of members of families with hyperactive children have diabetes, obesity, alcoholism, or all three. These are all sugar consumption problems. Unfortunately, it's often a child's dietary programming that results in their criminal behavior as an adult.

The treatment, however, is simple. *Dump the sugar.* Diets restricted in sugar have been demonstrated to decrease antisocial behavior, especially in males.

The hypoglycemic syndrome can be treated by the adoption of the keto-genic diet (see Chapter 3) that will, in up to 3 months, normalize insulin, blood sugar, and stress hormones. However, if you have been taking anti-depressant drugs, it will take longer, as the body needs to rebuild proper receptors (damaged by drugs) for the natural neurotransmitters derived from a ketogenic diet to normalize. You must withdraw from these drugs gradually under a doctor's supervision.

The Best Foods for People with Hypoglycemia

- Fruit. No more than two pieces per day. Because of its high fructose content, fruit should be consumed with other low-GI food, such as protein, and not consumed on its own.

- Green vegetables. You can eat as much as you want. However, pumpkins and sweet potatoes should be watched, as they are higher on the GI scale.

- Eggs and meats.

- Raw, unsalted seeds and nuts. Salted nuts are addictive, and you find yourself eating a lot more. These are not sufficient as a meal on their own.

- Low-GI bread and cereals without sugar added.

- Milk products such as cheese, yogurt, milk, and butter, only if you are not allergic or sensitive to them. If you are, try goat's milk, rice milk, soy milk, almond milk, hazelnut milk, or quinoa milk as alternatives.

- Basmati or whole grain brown rice.

- Raw, healthy oils (not used for cooking, preferably cold pressed and organic).

Dietary Supplements Recommended for Hypoglycemia

Most people with hypoglycemia will require some vitamin supplementation initially and should include a multi-B complex, chromium (to assist with food cravings), zinc, magnesium, vitamin D, and vitamin C. These are necessary for the synthesis of many other neurotransmitters in the brain, such as dopamine, norepinephrine, and acetylcholine. For example, if someone is deficient in vitamin B6 — a coenzyme involved in the conversion of tryptophan (found in chicken, eggs, fish, cheese) to serotonin — then this could be a factor in making them feel depressed (a good multivitamin should cover most of the required macronutrients).

If withdrawal symptoms from the high-sugar diet are unpleasant, two teaspoons of glycerine mixed in a glass of milk, or mixed with water and a dash of lemon juice, can be taken three times a day until the symptoms have passed. Glycerine is a vegetable extract that does not affect insulin levels or the pancreas and is a ready supply of energy to the brain. (Note: glycerol is the same as glycerine.)

Are You Getting Enough Fat?

We have become so fat-phobic as a society that most of us don't have enough fat in our diet. To get enough fats, we can either eat a heaped tablespoon of cold pressed seed oils or coconut oil every day (yum!) or we can eat oily fish such as sardines, trout, mackerel, herring, or tuna up to three times a week.

I would recommend supplementing concentrated oils. For omega-3, this means taking either concentrated fish oil capsules with eicosapentaenoic acid (EPA) and docosahexaenoic acid (DHA) or flaxseed oil capsules. Krill oil, like fish oil, contains these omega-3 fats; however, in fish oil, these omega-3 fats are found in the triglyceride form. In krill oil, they are found in a double-chain phospholipid structure.

The fats in human cell walls are in the phospholipid form. The phospholipid structure of the EPA and DHA in krill oil makes them much more absorbable. Krill oil also contains vitamin E, vitamin A, vitamin D, and astaxanthin, which is a potent antioxidant. The antioxidant potency of krill oil is, regarding ORAC (Oxygen Radical Absorbance Capacity) values, 48 times more potent than fish oil. The astaxanthin found in krill oil also provides excellent protection against ultraviolet light and UV-induced skin damage.

The recommended dose is 1,000 milligrams a day (two 500 mg capsules). This is based, in part, on clinical trials that showed benefits at this dose.

For omega-6, this means supplementing a source of gamma-linoleic acid (GLA). GLA is found in several plant-based oils, including Evening Primrose Oil (EPO), borage oil, and black currant seed oil. The recommended dose is three grams or four 750 mg capsules per day, for a 150-pound adult.

Summary

It's essential that we eat healthy to feed our brain. Eat as many green, leafy vegetables as you want. Eat dairy like cheese, milk, yogurt, and butter. And eat healthy fats, which can be found in sardines, salmon, beef, eggs, nuts, coconut oil, butter, sunflower oil, avocado, and olive oil.

I would recommend supplementing concentrated oils. For omega-3, this means taking either concentrated fish oil capsules with eicosapentaenoic acid (EPA) and docosahexaenoic acid (DHA) or flaxseed oil capsules. The recommended dose is 1,000 milligrams a day (two 500 mg capsules).

For omega-6, this means supplementing a source of gamma-linoleic acid (GLA). GLA is found in several plant-based oils, including evening primrose oil (EPO), The recommended dose is three grams or four 750 mg capsules per day

A high-potency multivitamin or B-complex vitamin is recommended. Make sure it contains about ten times (or 1,000 percent) of the recommended daily value for vitamins B1, B2, B3 and B6 since they play important roles in the synthesis of mood-regulating neurotransmitters, chromium (to assist with food cravings), zinc, magnesium, vitamin D, and vitamin C.

Depression and hypoglycemia have been linked to sugar consumption problems. So, dump the sugar — it's poison.

Chapter 10

Address
Your Stress

The brain uses feel-good transmitters called endorphins (opiods), in handling daily stress. When large amounts are needed to manage stress, the other transmitters become upset and create a chemical imbalance. We then begin to feel the pressure more acutely, and the sense of anxiety and urgency causes more stress. Harmful chemicals are released in our bodies that do damage and cause more stress. We call this vicious cycle the "stress cycle." The result is emotional fatigue, which can be experienced and felt like depression.

Over the years, researchers have gained insight into the long-term effects that stress has on physical and psychological health. Research suggests that prolonged stress contributes to brain changes that may contribute to addiction, anxiety, depression, high blood pressure, and the formation of artery-clogging deposits.

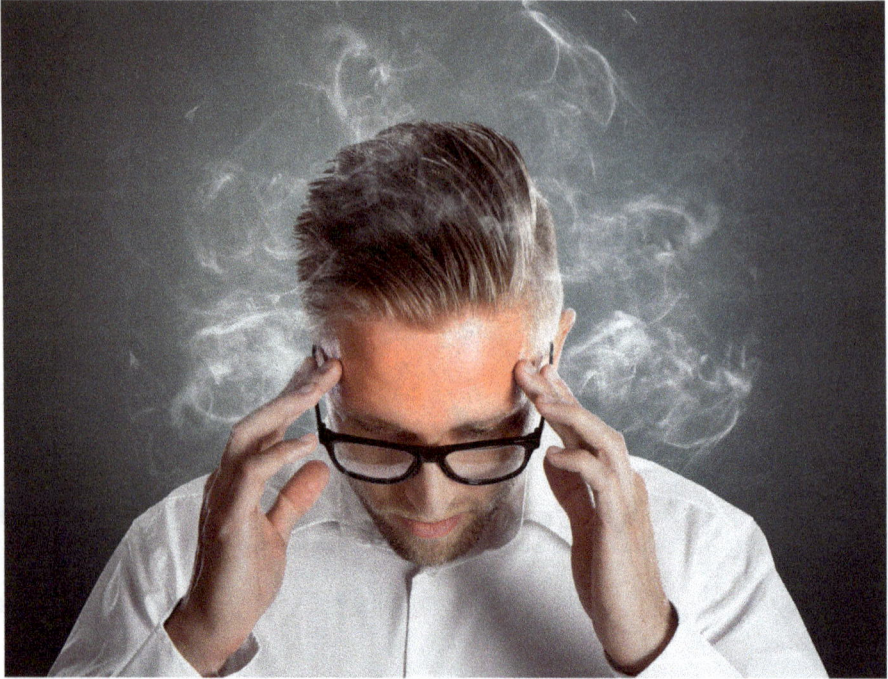

Recent research suggests that chronic stress may also contribute to weight issues and obesity, both through direct mechanisms (causing people to eat more) or indirectly (decreasing sleep and exercise).

Researchers estimate that stress contributes to as many as 80 percent of all the primary illnesses that include cancer, cardiovascular disease, metabolic and endocrine disease, skin disorders, and infectious ailments of all kinds.

Fortunately, people can learn techniques to counter the stress response.

How to Counter the Stress Response

Get enough sleep

Insomnia is a common problem that takes a toll on your mood, health, energy, and ability to function during the day. Do you struggle to get to sleep no matter how tired you are? Or do you wake up in the middle of the night and lie awake for hours, anxiously watching the clock?

Chronic insomnia can even contribute to serious health problems. Survey findings show that stress may be getting in the way of quality sleep. And sleep scientists agree that new guidelines are needed to consider the field's recent research and to find out why the average American is sleeping far less than they did in the past.

Several sleep studies have found that seven hours is the optimal amount of sleep — not eight, as was long believed — when it comes to certain cognitive and health markers, although many doctors question that conclusion.

Research also shows a link between sleep deprivation and Alzheimer's disease. Those studies showed a link in mice between sleep loss and brain plaques, a hallmark of Alzheimer's disease. Early evidence tentatively suggests the connection may work in both directions: Alzheimer's plaques disrupt sleep, and lack of sleep promotes Alzheimer's plaques.

Other recent research has shown that skimping on a full night's sleep, even by 20 minutes, impairs performance and memory the next day. And getting too much sleep — not just too little of it — is associated with health problems like diabetes, obesity, and cardiovascular disease and with higher rates of death. According to Dr. Shawn Youngstedt, a professor in the College of Nursing and Health Innovation at Arizona State University Phoenix, the lowest mortality and morbidity is with seven hours of sleep, and nine hours of sleep or more has been shown to be hazardous.

Popping a mineral may be the last thing you think about when you are feeling edgy or stressed. Calcium and magnesium will do the trick by relaxing muscle and nerve cells. A lack of these two minerals will leave you feeling nervous, irritable, and aggressive.

Magnesium

Magnesium is an essential nutrient that helps you relax. It's also commonly depleted by chronic stress

Magnesium not only relaxes your mind, but it also relaxes your muscles. Symptoms of deficiency include cramps, muscle aches, spasms, insomnia, and anxiety. Low levels are not uncommon in anxious people, and supplementation can often help. It is recommended you need about 500 mg of magnesium a day. Nuts and seeds are abundant in it, as are fruits and vegetables, especially dark green leafy vegetables like kale or spinach. I recommend eating these magnesium-rich foods every day and supplementing an additional 300 mg. But, if you were particularly anxious, and can't sleep, increase your supplementation to 500 mg in the evening.

Calcium

Because calcium is needed for healthy brain function, calcium deficiency can lead to changes in your behavior. Anxiety, jitters, depression and irritability are common in those with calcium deficiency. The symptoms may be subtle at times, but you will get a sense that something isn't right. Low blood calcium can result in lethargy, muscle cramping, numb fingers and toes, and heart palpitations.

Calcium also protects our bodies from cancer, high blood pressure, and diabetes. Many people over the age of 50 don't get enough calcium in their diets, and the body doesn't produce calcium on its own, so supplementing is recommended. For preventive measures, 1000 mg of calcium and 50[mcg] of vitamin D is a combination that works (vitamin D is essential to absorb the calcium). But you should also increase your intake of calcium-rich foods in addition to supplementing.

Calcium can be found in a variety of foods, including dairy products like milk, yogurt, and cheese; dark green leafy vegetables like spinach, kale, and broccoli; and fish with edible soft bones, like sardines and canned salmon.

To begin a new path towards healthier sleep and a healthier lifestyle, start by assessing your own individual needs and habits. See how you respond to different amounts of sleep. Pay careful attention to your mood, energy, and health after a poor night's sleep versus a good one. Ask yourself, "How often do I get a good night's sleep?" Like good diet and exercise, sleep is a critical component to overall health.

Most importantly, make sleep a priority. You must schedule sleep like any other daily activity — put it on your to-do list and cross it off every night. But don't make it the thing you do only after everything else is done — stop everything else and stay on schedule.

To pave the way for better sleep, follow these simple yet effective, Healthy sleep tips:

- Stick to a sleep schedule, even on weekends.
- Practice a relaxing bedtime ritual.
- Exercise daily.
- Evaluate your bedroom to ensure ideal temperature, sound, and light.

- Sleep on a comfortable mattress and pillow.
- Beware of hidden sleep thieves like alcohol and coffee.
- Turn off all electronics before bed — especially that phone.
- Supplement magnesium [500mg in the evening] and calcium 1000mg.

Talk to someone

If managing work, family, or school is driving your stress levels through the roof, talking face to face with someone who cares about you is a great way to relieve stress and stop you from rehashing worries when it's time to sleep. The person doesn't need to be able to fix your problems; they just need to be an attentive, non-judgmental listener — this is called the buffering theory.

The buffering theory is that people who enjoy close relationships with family and friends receive emotional support that indirectly helps to sustain them at times of stress and crisis.

Exercise

People can use exercise to stifle the buildup of stress in several ways. Exercise, even just taking a brisk walk shortly after feeling stressed, not only deepens breathing, but also helps relieve muscle tension. Movement therapies such as yoga, tai chi, and qi gong combine fluid movements with deep breathing and mental focus, all of which can induce calm.

Breathe

We all know how to breathe, but getting the most from each breath during a stressful time can relax your muscles, decrease your heart rate, and eventually lower your blood pressure. Try these different techniques when you have the time and space to do so. As you become more comfortable with these exercises (or other activities that help you relax), incorporate them into your everyday routines.

Take yourself off to a quiet place — even locking yourself in the bathroom if need be. To start, inhale through your nose for a count of four, hold for a count of four, then exhale through your nose for a count of four. (Inhaling and exhaling through the nose adds a natural resistance to the breath.) This is a great technique that is especially effective before bed.

Much like counting sheep, if you're having trouble falling asleep, this breathing exercise can help take your mind off racing thoughts or whatever might be distracting you. Once you get familiar with the exercise, inhale for a count of seven, hold for seven and exhale for seven.

Power posing

Power posing is positioning your body into a posture of confidence, even when you don't feel confident. It can affect cortisol and testosterone levels in the brain, and it might even have an impact on our chances for success. You can feel the changes in your anxiety levels and stress levels after only two minutes. Find a quiet place (even if it turns out to be the tiny room containing the toilet, an elevator, or in a closed room behind your desk and stand with your legs shoulder-width apart. Hold yourself tall. Raise your arms above your head in a victory pose. The victory pose is very empowering. Hold this position for two minutes.

Power posing for pitching an idea: Rest your feet on the table, clasp your hands behind your head, and lean back.

Power posing for conducting an interview: Rest your arm on the back of your chair, keep your knees apart, and recline.

Power posing for a chit chat with your boss; Puff out your chest, plant your hands on your hips and stand with feet hip-width apart.

Adrenal Fatigue Syndrome

Flight or fight hormones. They are involved in producing over 50 hormones that drive almost every bodily function, many of which are essential for life. Adrenal fatigue is a condition where the body and adrenal glands can't keep up with the tremendous amount of daily stress many people experience.

Adrenal communication with the hypothalamus and the pituitary gland in a system known as the hypothalamus-pituitary-adrenal axis (HPA axis) stimulates the adrenal gland to make and release cortisol. Cortisol is a hormone that plays several important roles in the body. It helps with the body's use of fats, proteins, and carbohydrates. It suppresses inflammation, regulates blood pressure, increases blood sugar, and can decrease bone formation. This hormone also controls the sleep/wake cycle. It is released during times of stress to help your body cope and get an extra boost.

The problem with adrenal fatigue is that you store more fat around your stomach area, and this is stubborn fat to lose. The visceral fat (belly fat) and stress increase as you age. All stress is accumulative. You are like a sponge. You soak up stress from childhood onwards.

The brain is also affected by the adrenals. If you can't switch off the brain and you worry constantly, it can affect your memory. Why am I going down the stairs? I forgot what I was going to do. Where are my keys? Where did I put them?

This memory is affected by adrenal fatigue. Your patience goes out the window. Tolerance levels go out the window. Logic goes out the window. Sleep is also affected by adrenals, as you cannot switch off your repetitive thoughts or racing mind. We have a circadian rhythm that requires four types of sleep every night. Every 90 minutes, we go through this cycle of light sleep and deep sleep. It's during the deep sleep that human growth hormone (HGH) is released in the body and burns fat. If you are not getting the appropriate amount of sleep, you are not burning fat.

You will get salt cravings (chips and cheeses, etc). Stress uses minerals like sodium, potassium, and magnesium with the adrenal. This can cause cravings. You need to increase your salt increase with sea salt or mineral salt, not junk food.

Another thing that happens with the adrenal is your urine starts to become acidic. This is because you lose beneficial acids with adrenals. So, now you crave acid! You start craving lemons and other citrus fruit. Consuming apple cider vinegar or lemon in water will help replace the acids.

Adrenal glands sit just above your kidneys, which are in the middle of your lower back area. You have one adrenal gland for each kidney. Why are they located next to the kidneys? Because they have a strong influence on your kidney function (as well as many other things).

An easy way to understand the structure of the adrenal glands is to compare them to a fruit, like an avocado. There are three distinct layers that you need to know, and I will briefly describe each one. Further on, I will also go into detail on the functions that each layer performs.

The capsule

The adipose capsule is a protective layer of fat that surrounds each adrenal gland. Think of this as being like the skin of the avocado. Although not strictly a part of the adrenal glands themselves, the primary function of this layer is to enclose and protect each of the adrenals.

The cortex

You might compare this layer to the flesh of an avocado. It comprises around 80 percent of the volume of the adrenal gland, and it surrounds the medulla, which lies in the center.

The cortex and the medulla have very separate roles, although there is some interaction between them. There are two functions that the cortex typically performs.

The first is the production of dehydroepiandrosterone (DHEA) and other sex hormones. This occurs in the innermost layer of the cortex, the zona reticularis. Hormones like DHEA and DHEA-S are produced and secreted as needed. In men, these hormones can be converted into testosterone within the testes (although, the testes can also produce testosterone directly from cholesterol without the adrenal glands). In women, the adrenal glands are the primary source of these androgens ("male" sex hormones), and so they play a much more important role.

The second function of the cortex controls our production of cortisol, which is performed by the middle section of the cortex, or the zona fasciculate. Cortisol and its related compounds are essential hormones that we literally cannot live without. They control our waking and sleeping cycle, they suppress inflammation, they help us generate energy from non-carbohydrate foods, and they even regulate our blood pressure.

The medulla

The medulla helps you cope with emotional and physical stress. The main hormones secreted by the medulla include norepinephrine (noradrenaline) and epinephrine (adrenaline). These hormones are capable of increasing the heart rate, increasing blood flow to the brain and muscles, assisting in sugar metabolism, and relaxing muscles. They control the squeezing of the blood vessels, which helps maintain blood pressure and increase it in response to stress. Like several other hormones produced by the adrenal glands, epinephrine and norepinephrine are often activated in stressful situations when your body needs additional resources and energy to cope with significant strain.

There are ways you can support this important part of your endocrine system, to heal, and feel whole again.

Here are the best ways to fight adrenal exhaustion.

1. Rid your diet of excess sugar and processed grains. These are very hard on the adrenal glands. Eating excess sugar and starches will cause blood sugar to spike and insulin to come to the rescue due to excess glucose in the bloodstream. Blood sugar then drops, causing the adrenals to work to bring levels back up. When you are suffering from fatigued adrenal glands, cortisol levels drop and make it difficult to maintain normal blood sugar levels. People with adrenal fatigue tend to have low blood sugar. Low blood sugar is the other stressful situation that can further tax your adrenal glands.

2. Add healthy fats. Coconut oil, olives, organic olive oil, and clarified butter all significantly support adrenal health. Some of these oils will also lower belly fat, which screams "adrenal fatigue."

3. Get more sleep. Seven to eight hours a night is vital. Even if you don't feel tired, try turning off all electronics (cell phones, computers, tablets, etc.) and close your eyes in an entirely dark room before 10 p.m. Even if you don't fall asleep and stay asleep, you are lowering your stress levels and retraining your body to sleep when it should be sleeping.

4. Breathe right. Deep, controlled breathing has astoundingly positive effects on adrenal health and your overall stress.

5. Eat your greens and brightly colored vegetables. There is sound evidence that eating the proper nutrition consistently can help the adrenals in a profound way.

6. Sip on green tea. Organic green tea has high levels of healthful phytochemicals ,which support the adrenal glands. Matcha green tea is the best.

7. Do your best to eliminate stress. I know, easier said than done, but adding just one session of yoga, meditation or tai chi a week can help greatly with overly-stressed adrenal glands. And don't forget your breathing exercises.

8. Eating a high-fat high protein breakfast sets your day up nicely. Opt for an omelet with three eggs and cooked in butter or coconut oil.

9. Consume natural salt like Himalayan sea salt. Natural salts contain many trace minerals that help to support the adrenals. Adrenal fatigue reduces the production of the hormone aldosterone, which helps regulate salt in the body. Many people feel better when consuming adequate levels of real salt.

10. Connect with the earth. Be sure to practice grounding by placing as much of your body (just bare feet is sufficient) on the ground as possible. When you walk barefoot on the Earth, do you notice you feel better? Your immune system functions at optimum levels when you are in direct contact with the ground whether it be grass, dirt or sand due to the Earth's electrons directly in touch with your body, bringing it to the same electrical potential as the earth and promoting favorable physiological changes that promote optimum health. The ultimate antioxidant and anti-inflammatory benefits are emerging and an improved balance of the autonomic nervous system is notable.

11. Limit the use of stimulants like coffee when you are suffering from adrenal fatigue.

12. Don't overtrain at the gym. Excessive cardio or endurance training is extremely hard on the adrenals. When you are suffering from many of the symptoms listed in this chapter, it might be better to practice a more relaxing form of exercise.

13. Eat your mushrooms. Mushrooms have stress-relieving properties, and they boost overall levels of health.

14. Add herbs to your diet. Ashwagandha, ginseng, and astragalus are great examples of herbs that support the body in stress relief and overall adrenal health.

By practicing one or all of these natural adrenal-rescuing habits, you should start feeling more rested, healthy, and energetic over time.

Summary

You can recover from Adrenal fatigue. It is not easy and there are no quick fixes, but the advice in this chapter covers the big picture and will see you on the road to recovery. The breathing exercises are important and can calm your nervous system. Deep, controlled breathing has astoundingly positive effects on adrenal health and your overall stress.

Get more Sleep, 7- 8 hrs a night is vital; Add healthy fats — coconut oil, ghee, olives, organic olive oil, and clarified butter; Eat your greens and brightly colored vegetables; Exercise daily., but don't over-train at the Gym — excessive cardio or endurance training is extremely hard on the adrenals. Most of all, Be patient.

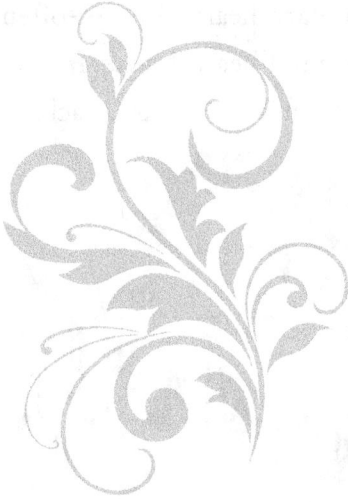

Chapter 11

Reducing Your Risk of Heart Disease

Y ou have a 50 percent chance of dying from heart or artery disease. That is pretty grim news. But take heart! The good news is you can completely prevent this disease. There is nothing natural about dying from heart disease. Many cultures do not experience a high incidence of strokes or heart attacks. France has the lowest ranking per capita, followed by Italy.

What is Heart Disease?

The term heart disease covers numerous problems that affect the heart. They can affect the heart in several ways, but basically they disrupt the pumping action of the heart. Coronary heart disease—often simply called heart disease—is the main form of heart disease. It is a disorder of the blood vessels of the heart that can lead to heart attack.

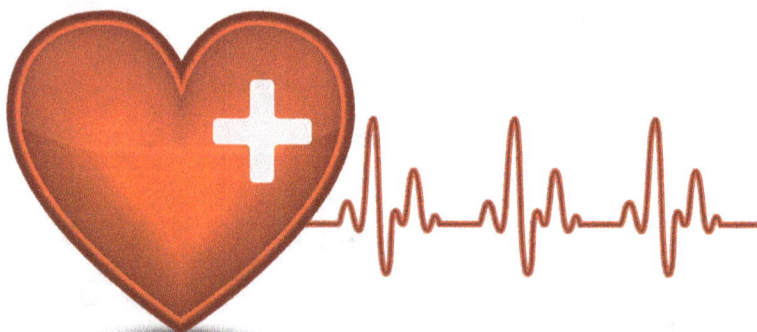

The basic cause of heart disease is the accumulation of fatty deposits on the walls of the arteries. These fatty deposits take years to build up in the artery walls in a process medically known as atherosclerosis. The fatty deposits called plaques or atheroma are made up of many substances including cholesterol. Over time, the artery may become so narrow that it can't deliver enough blood oxygen to your heart, especially when you are exerting yourself. This can lead to angina, during which you will feel pain or discomfort in your chest.

Preventing and Reversing Heart Disease

So, how do you prevent, or even reverse, cardiovascular heart disease? Combining exercise and diet, taking the right supplements, and improving your lifestyle has shown to be far more effective than taking prescription drugs — without all the side effects.

Exaggerated vs. real risk factors

There's a difference between real risk factors and exaggerated risk factors designed to sell prescription drugs. Most people have been lead to believe that cholesterol levels in the blood reflect eating fat or cholesterol. This isn't true. Cholesterol is produced by the body when your blood sugar and insulin levels rise; losing blood sugar control is a primary driver of high cholesterol, and controlling your blood sugar with the ketogenic diet is the main way to reduce it.

A study published in the *British Medical Journal* shows that your homocysteine level, found through a simple blood test, predicts the risk of death from cardiovascular disease in older people better than any conventional measure of risk — including blood pressure, smoking, or cholesterol.

Reducing fat in your diet doesn't reduce heart disease risk unless you replace animal fats with fish. However, if you replace fat with carbs, which is what most so-called low-fat foods do, your risk of heart disease can go up. Also, reducing your cholesterol intake by eating fewer eggs makes absolutely no difference to your risk of heart disease.

Lower your cholesterol

Niacin (vitamin B3) in high doses of 500 mg, is by far the most effective cholesterol-lowering substance because it lowers the "lousy" low-density lipoprotein (LDL) and it raises the "healthy" HDL high-density lipoprotein (HDL). It also reverses arterial thickening (atherosclerosis) and the risk of cardiovascular events. Niacin is usually recommended at a dose of 1,000 mg a day (500 mg twice a day), although slightly better results are achieved with 2,000 mg a day.

Lower your blood pressure

Studies show that you can lower high blood pressure with magnesium, vitamin B, and vitamin C. High blood pressure is a risk factor for a heart attack and also an indicator of cardiovascular disease because it either means the arteries are already becoming restricted or are harder, possibly due to muscular contraction. Magnesium helps muscles relax. A study, published in *Angiology* shows that magnesium lowers high blood pressure by about 10 percent, and research published in *Scientific American* demonstrates that magnesium reduces cholesterol and triglycerides as well.

A lot of us are deficient in magnesium. The richest source of this mineral is dark green vegetables, nuts, and seeds (especially pumpkin seeds). These are all good foods to eat, but if you have high blood pressure or any type of heart disease, I recommend supplementing with 300 mg of magnesium a day. A good multivitamin might give you 150 mg, so you'll need at least an extra 150 mg. It is cheap, safe, and highly effective.

Vitamin C also works. A meta-analysis of 29 trials found that a mere 500 mg of vitamin C a day lowers high blood pressure by five points in eight weeks. This study, published in the *American Journal of Clinical Nutrition*, confirms this important effect of vitamin C.

Get your essential fats

Omega-3 fats cut your risk of a heart attack in half, so try to get three servings of oily fish a week. Two long-term studies published in *The Lancet* comparing the effects of giving cholesterol-lowering statin drugs or omega-3 fish oils to heart-failure patients found that those taking one gram a day of omega-3 fats cut their premature death risk by nine percent and cut their risk of admission to hospital by eight percent compared to the placebo. Those taking statin drugs had no reduction in risk.

The UK's National Institute for Clinical Excellence recommends all doctors prescribe one gram of fish oil a day for a six-month period to patients who have had a heart attack. The American Heart Association (AHA) has recommended that all adults eat fish, particularly fatty fish, at least twice a week, as well as omega-3 fats.

Another essential fat for reducing heart disease risk is vitamin D. Exactly how vitamin D protects the heart is not clear yet, but one way is probably by keeping the endothelium (the very delicate lining of blood vessels) flexible, making you less likely to suffer high blood pressure.

Symptoms of a Heart Attack in Men

You are more likely to experience a heart attack if you're a man. Men also have heart attacks earlier in life compared to women. If you have a family history of heart disease or a history of high blood pressure, cigarette smoking, obesity, high blood cholesterol, or other risk factors, your chances of having a heart attack are even higher.

Symptoms of a heart attack in men include:

- Standard chest pain that feels like "an elephant" is sitting on your chest, with a squeezing sensation that may come and go or remain constant and intense
- Upper body pain or discomfort, including arms, left shoulder, back, neck, jaw, or stomach
- Rapid or irregular heartbeat

- Stomach discomfort that feels like indigestion
- Shortness of breath, which may leave you feeling like you can't get enough air, even when you're resting
- Dizziness or feeling like you're going to pass out
- Breaking out in a cold sweat

It's important to remember, however, that each heart attack is different. Your symptoms may not fit these descriptions. Trust your instincts if you think something is wrong.

Symptoms of a Heart Attack in Women

In recent decades, scientists have realized that heart attack symptoms can be quite different in women than in men. Heart attack symptoms for women can be subtle and are not always easy to diagnose without a blood test and assessment by medical professionals, and heart trouble can easily be confused with other ailments, like indigestion.

Forty percent of women won't experience the typical crushing chest pain, but most experience symptoms such as shortness of breath or unusual fatigue for weeks or even months before a cardiac event. They are also more likely to experience non-chest pain symptoms such as:

- Unusual fatigue lasting for several days
- Sudden severe fatigue
- Sleep disturbances
- Anxiety
- Light-headedness
- Shortness of breath
- Indigestion or gas-like pain
- Upper back, shoulder, or throat pain

- Jaw pain or pain that spreads up to your jaw
- Pressure or pain in the center of your chest, which may spread to your arm

Women, particularly between the ages of 45 and 65, are more likely to have abnormalities of the function of the small arteries — blood vessels so small that you do not even see them on the traditional diagnostic angiogram. And they are also more likely to be falsely reassured by medical professionals that it's perhaps a bad case of indigestion, when, in fact, there really is a problem. If you have unusual pain, then you should always get medical attention. Call for an ambulance and don't worry about being embarrassed if it turns out to be a false alarm. Or get a family member or a friend to drive you to the hospital. Never try to drive yourself.

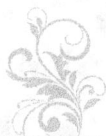

Summary

You have a 50 percent chance of dying from heart or artery disease. If you want to prevent this, you need to improve your diet and lifestyle. Take control of your blood sugar with the ketogenic diet. Lower your high blood pressure with 300 mg of magnesium and 500 mg of vitamin C a day. Lower your cholesterol with niacin (vitamin B3) in high doses of 1,000 mg a day (500 mg twice a day). Get your essential fats through fatty fish at least twice a week. And don't forget to exercise!

Chapter 12

Dementia and Alzheimer's

A recent research study found that age-related decline could start as early as 45. The good news is that some promising research indicates that risk of dementia and Alzheimer's could be reduced in the initial stages by a comprehensive optimum nutrition approach. Many people wrongly assume that failing memory and concentration is an inevitable part of the aging process. It doesn't have to be.

When it comes to the brain, size does matter. The bigger the brain, the better the brain. We can grow our brain bigger. The solutions are at our fingertips. There is a lot you can do *today* to ensure that you don't get the shriveling of the brain that gradually leads from memory decline to Alzheimer's disease.

Brain shrinkage starts, for many, in their 40's. So, the prevention must start now, not just later in life. The stress it brings, both to the sufferer and their family, is enormous. With the baby boomers' ever-ageing population, the prediction is that by 2030, 20 percent of people over 65 will have dementia or Alzheimer's disease. The first symptoms are depression, irritability, confusion, and forgetfulness.

Alzheimer's is a complex disease with several risk factors. Some, like your genetics and age, are outside your control. But many others are within your sphere of influence. And these can be quite impressive when it comes to brain health. The six pillars of a brain-healthy, Alzheimer's prevention lifestyle are:

- **Regular exercise;** helps prevent or manage a broad range of health problems and concerns: strokes, metabolic syndrome, type 2 diabetes, depression, many types of cancer, arthritis and falls. Do you want to have more energy, feel better and add more years to your life? By just exercising? The benefits of regular physical exercise and activity to your health are hard to ignore. Everyone benefits from exercise, regardless of age, sex or physical ability. Aim for at least 150 minutes[less than 3 hours] per week of moderate-intensity exercise, or 75 minutes[just over an hour] per week of vigorous exercise.

- **Healthy diet and supplementation:** A balanced, healthy diet often provides your body with essential vitamins and minerals, but taking dietary supplements on top of your healthy diet may prove beneficial in ensuring your body gets all the required nutrients it needs daily. Your body breaks down proteins, carbohydrates, and fats from your meal, and absorbs other nutrients from the food. There are at least 30 vitamins, minerals, and dietary components that your body needs but cannot manufacture on its own in sufficient amounts.

- **Mental stimulation:** Mental exercise keeps your memory, and mental skills in tone, much like exercise does to muscle. Continuing to learn new things creates and maintains connections between brain cells you have spent the first half of your life building. No matter what your age, exercising your brain can help reduce your risk of developing dementia, doing brain exercises like jigsaw puzzles, crosswords, word puzzles or board games.

- **Stress management:** Stress management is imperative. Learning how to breathe properly is one of the best stress management techniques. Remember the breathing exercises in chapter 10? Take yourself off to a quiet place and breath.

- **An active social life:** Staying socially active appears to help lessen age-related challenges people often experience later in life. Living socially active lives and prioritizing social activity are associated with higher late-life satisfaction and less severe declines toward the end of life. A socially engaged lifestyle often involves cognitive stimulation and physical activity, which in turn may protect against cognitive and physical decline, maintaining wellbeing later in life.

- **Quality sleep:** Research shows a link between sleep deprivation and Alzheimer's disease. Those studies showed a link in mice between sleep loss and brain plaques, a hallmark of Alzheimer's disease. [More in below]. 8 simple ways to help you sleep: Read a magazine or book by a soft light, listen to some soft music, take a warm bath, wind down with a favorite hobby, do some easy stretches and dim the lights in the hour leading up to bed.

Quality Sleep

All six of the pillars are important, but we need to discuss quality sleep in a little more depth. Sleep problems are common in people who have symptomatic Alzheimer's disease, but scientists have recently begun to suspect that they also may be an indicator of early disease. This finding is the first to connect early Alzheimer's disease and sleep disruption in humans.

For the study, researchers recruited 145 volunteers from the University's Charles F. and Joanne Knight Alzheimer's Disease Research Center. All the volunteers were 45 to 75 years old and cognitively normal when they enrolled. As a part of other research at the center, scientists had analyzed samples of the volunteers' spinal fluids for markers of Alzheimer's disease. The samples showed that 32 participants had preclinical Alzheimer's disease, meaning they were likely to have amyloid plaques present in their brains but were not yet cognitively impaired.

Participants kept daily sleep diaries for two weeks, noting the time they went to bed and got up, the number of naps taken on the previous day, and other sleep-related information. The researchers tracked the participants' activity levels using sensors worn on the wrist that detected the wearer's movements. "Most people don't move when they're asleep," says author Yo-El Ju, MD, assistant professor of neurology, "and we developed a way to use the data we collected as a marker for whether a person was asleep or awake. This lets us monitor sleep efficiency, which is a measure of how much time in bed is spent asleep."

Participants who had preclinical Alzheimer's disease had poorer sleep efficiency (80.4 percent) than people without. "When we looked specifically at the worst sleepers, those with a sleep efficiency lower than 75 percent, they were more than five times more likely to have preclinical Alzheimer's disease than good sleepers," Ju says.

Therefore, it's important to make sleep a priority. Schedule sleep like any other daily activity: Put it on your to-do list, and cross it off every night. Don't wait until you finish other tasks, either. Stay on track.

Homocysteine

Forget your blood pressure, your cholesterol, even your weight! There is one factor that can determine whether you will live long and healthy or die young. It's *homocysteine*.

There is substantial evidence proving that raised homocysteine levels both predict risk and can cause the kind of brain damage seen in Alzheimer's. One of the best ways to prevent Alzheimer's is to lower your homocysteine.

What is homocysteine? And why haven't we been hearing more about it? Homocysteine is a non-protein amino acid produced by the body and found in the blood. Ideally, it should be present in low quantities. However, if you are not optimally nourished, homocysteine can accumulate in the blood and increase the risk of over 50 diseases, including strokes, heart attacks, diabetes, certain cancers, depression, and Alzheimer's disease.

One in two people have high homocysteine levels — that's the bad news. The good news is that this important risk factor can be reversed in two weeks. Evidence indicates that if you can lower your homocysteine score, you will significantly reduce your risk of getting Alzheimer's disease. Homocysteine is strongly linked to damage in the brain. Doctors and colleagues at Tokyo University conducted brain scans on 153 senior citizens and checked them against each's homocysteine level. The evidence was crystal clear — the higher the homocysteine, the greater the damage to the brain.

Homocysteine itself isn't bad. Your body naturally turns it into two beneficial substances — glutathione (the body's most important antioxidant) and SAMe (a vital type of intelligent nutrient for the brain and body). The trouble is this: if you don't have optimal amounts of B vitamins in your diet, the enzymes that turn homocysteine into these beneficial substances don't work well enough. Your homocysteine can't be converted, so your levels of it rise dangerously.

New evidence is emerging that many mental health problems, as well as heart disease, cancer, and diabetes, are linked to excessive homocysteine, usually from related inflammation.

Alzheimer's is certainly an inflammatory disease, but autism, depression, Parkinson's disease, and possibly schizophrenia can be as well. We are beginning to learn that inflammation upsets the brain as much as the body and that homocysteine may be the best indicator. For example, 52 percent of depressed patients have high homocysteine. It has also been found to be very common in schizophrenia. Having a high homocysteine level doubles your risk for Alzheimer's disease.

What can you do to lower risk? It can easily be done with the right combination of nutrients, dietary changes, and lifestyle changes.

- Supplement with a high-strength multivitamin every day. At least 25 mg of the main B vitamins (B vitamins are so fundamental to our mental health and wellbeing they should be prescribed to everybody).

- Add 200 mcg of folate and 10 mcg each of B12 and B6 — plus A, D, and E, and the minerals manganese, selenium, chromium, and zinc.

- Increase your intake of omega-3 with fish oil supplements and by eating more fish.

- Exercise more, eat vegetables and greens, limit alcohol, stop smoking, and reduce your stress.

A combination of these factors could eliminate one-third of Alzheimer's cases.

Vitamin C

Vitamin C does more than just prevent a cold. According to a new study from Weill Cornell Medicine investigators, high levels of vitamin C have killed certain kinds of cancers in cell cultures of mice. The findings suggest that scientists could one-day harness vitamin C to develop targeted treatments.

Vitamin C is essential for the body and the brain. Vitamin C supplements can improve memory, IQ, and other mental functions, especially in people with low levels of vitamin C.

This isn't surprising considering vitamin C is involved in making neurotransmitters, the chemicals that affect our mind and mood. Our bodies can't make or store vitamin C, so we must receive it every day through food and drinks and, if necessary, supplements. Getting the right amount of vitamin C is vital for good health because it has been shown to reduce both depression and schizophrenia when taken in much larger amounts than recommended.

Vitamin C is involved in making the neurotransmitters serotonin and noradrenaline, which affect our mood. It also helps protect us against many health problems, including age-related macular degeneration, cancer, asthma, the common cold, high blood pressure, heart disease, and osteoarthritis.

It is also an antioxidant that protects our bodies' cells (including brain cells) from damage and helps us fight diseases. It assists muscle function — helping make collagen (connective tissue) — and assists the growth and repair of the body's tissues, like wound healing and repairing and maintaining bones, gums, and teeth. And it is a natural antihistamine, which prevents the release of the chemical histamine in the body.

Some studies show that people who suffer mental health issues require vitamin C and are frequently deficient. And many of these same studies illustrate how higher amounts of vitamin C in the bloodstream can boost brain function at all ages and protect against age-related brain degeneration, including Alzheimer's and strokes.

Researchers at the University of Sydney in Australia studied 117 senior citizens. The study found that those who took vitamin C supplements were 40 percent less likely to have severe brain function problems compared to those who didn't take vitamin C. This was true regardless of education level. When supplement takers also ate a high vitamin C diet, the chance of mental decline dropped to 32 percent.

A Swiss study of people aged 65 to 94 showed that those with the highest blood levels of vitamin C did better on memory tests than those with low concentrations.

How much vitamin C should we receive daily? Countries and organizations differ regarding how much vitamin C they recommend. Here are some recommendations for adults.

The World Health Organization recommends 45 mg per day. The United Kingdom's Food Standards Agency (FSA) recommends 40 mg per day. The U.S. Department of Health & Human Services and Health Canada both recommend 90 mg per day. I recommend up to 1200mg per day. You can never have too much.

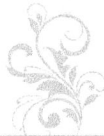

Summary

Alzheimer's is a complex disease with several risk factors. Some are outside your control, but many others are within your sphere of influence. To lower your risk of Alzheimer's, you should exercise regularly, keep an active social life, manage your stress, get plenty of mental stimulation, get seven to eight hours of quality sleep every night, and maintain a healthy diet.

Another way to lower your risk can be done by taking a daily, high-strength multivitamin to lower your homocysteine levels. The multivitamin should have at least 25 mg of the main B vitamins, 200 mcg of folate, and 10 mcg each of B12 and B6. Clinical studies have shown that the B vitamins not only correct homocysteine but can also increase life expectancy by seven to eight years. The multivitamin should also have A, D, and E and the minerals manganese, selenium, chromium, and zinc. You should also take vitamin C supplements to improve your memory, IQ, and other mental functions (1200 to 2000 mg a day) and increase your intake of omega-3 with fish oil supplements and by eating more fish.

The next chapter deals with helping yourself to maintain a calm approach to life — this will also help your brain.

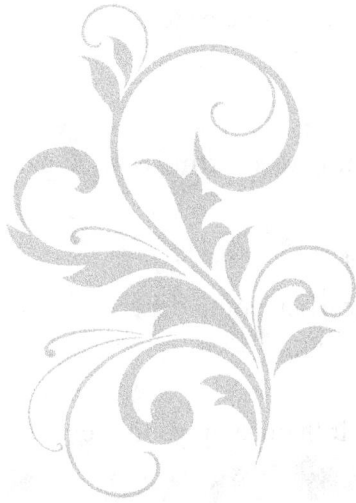

Chapter 13

Exercise

Ha — you thought you were going to get away without that, didn't you? Well, exercise is too powerful not to have on your side. Exercise unlocks the door to many improvements, as well as keeping the weight off. Regardless of what you do, regular exercise and physical activity is the path to proper health and wellbeing.

Exercise…

- Burns fat
- Builds muscle
- Eases stress and anxiety
- Lowers your risk of heart disease
- Lowers cholesterol

- Improves your immune system and helps to fight the common cold and flu
- Helps you sleep better
- Prevents chronic pain including osteoarthritis, back pain, and joint pain
- Prevents cancer and diabetes
- Improves your brains linkages, banishing depression and strengthening your mental health.

These benefits will have a profound influence on your later years.

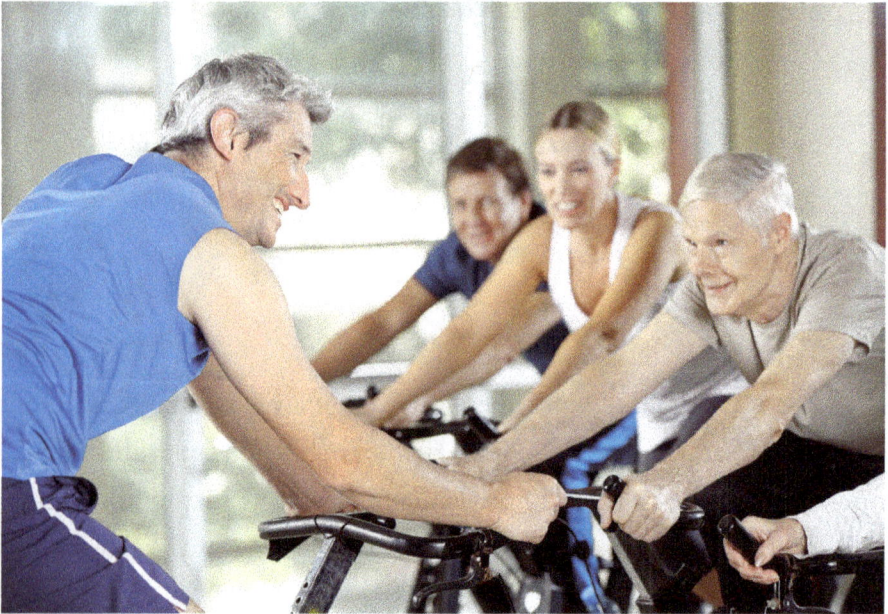

High-Intensity Exercise

There is ever-mounting research showing that the most beneficial form of exercise is short bursts of high-intensity exercise. Not only does it debunk regular cardio as the most effective and efficient form of exercise, but also provides remarkable health benefits you cannot get from regular aerobics.

Human growth hormone

High-intensity exercise has a tremendous boost in human growth hormone (HGH), hailed as the youth and fitness hormone. HGH is a synergistic, foundational biochemical that promotes muscle and effectively burns excessive fat. Unfortunately, once you hit your 30s, your levels of HGH begin to drop dramatically, a condition known as age-related growth hormone deficiency, or somatopause.

As your HGH levels decrease, your levels of insulin-like growth factor 1 (IGF-1) also decrease, which is another important factor that affects your body's aging process. This is why it is so important to boost your levels of HGH as you age. The longer your body can produce higher levels of HGH, the longer you will likely experience robust health and strength.

High-intensity interval training workouts help your body produce HGH naturally because they engage your fast twitch and super-fast twitch muscle fibers. These benefits are something you simply can't get from traditional, aerobic endurance training. We'll explore some of these exercises later in the chapter.

Telomere shortening

Another profound benefit of high-intensity training is the reduction of age-related telomere shortening. Studies have found that high-intensity exercises have a profound effect on the aging process of your cells. Your body is made up of more than 10 trillion cells. One theory states that you age because your cells age. Therefore, you can control your aging if you control the aging process of your cells. This is where stopping age-related telomere shortening comes in.

To learn what a telomere is, you must first know the typical structure of a cell. Every cell has a nucleus, which has gene-containing chromosomes. The chromosome is made up of two "arms," with each arm containing a single molecule DNA — this is a string of beads made up of units called bases.

Every DNA molecule is about 100 million bases long. The telomere is located at the tip of each chromosome arm. Every time your cells divide, starting at the moment of conception, your telomeres shorten. If you unravel the chromosome tip at the date of conception, your telomere will stretch to 15,000 bases long. Once your telomeres have been reduced to about 5,000 bases, you will mostly die of old age.

There is a certain intrinsic rate of telomere shortening that occurs just to keep you alive. However, telomere shortening is accelerated by factors like free radical exposure, trans fats, obesity, smoking, and other toxins.

Originally, telomere shortening was believed to be unaffected by healthy eating habits or exercise. But now, researchers have discovered a direct association between reduced telomere shortening in your later years and high-intensity-type exercises, like Peak Fitness.

This is very exciting because the prospect of being able to reduce telomere shortening —essentially stopping the cellular aging process that eventually kills you — is one of the most promising anti-aging strategies known to date. And it can begin with proper high-intensity exercises found in the Peak Fitness routine.

Peak Fitness

Peak Fitness is a high-intensity exercise program that is designed to increase your body's ability to produce HGH. Here is the basic rundown of the routine:

1. Warm up for four minutes.

2. Exercise as hard and fast as you can for 30 seconds. You should be puffing and panting for breath and feel like you couldn't possibly do anymore. I find it better to use lower resistance and higher repetitions to increase the heart rate.

3. Recovery for 90 seconds, moving at a much slower pace. Lowering the resistance every time you rest and then increasing it is sometimes difficult to get right, so just slow to a speed that allows your breathing to return to subnormal.

4. Repeat the high-intensity exercise seven more times — all the way to eight.

This is what I like about Peak Fitness. Short and sweet! I can't say I look forward to doing the routine for 20 minutes because it's so intense, but what I do love are the benefits. These 20-minute exercises only two or three times weekly can:

- Improve muscle tone
- Improve athletic speed and performance
- Improve your ability to achieve your fitness goals much faster
- Decrease body fat
- Firm skin
- Reduce wrinkles.

Remember, it's completely different from one person to another. You need to start out at a pace that suits you and build on that every week. Depending on your level of fitness currently, you may reach your anabolic threshold by walking at a quick pace, while others may need to perform at a higher speed to get the same effect. When you are first starting, you may only be able to do three or four reps, but as I said just keep adding more reps until you are doing the full eight.

Studies have shown that 12 weeks of high-intensity interval training not only can result in significant reductions in total abdominal, trunk, and visceral fat but also can give you significant increases in fat-free mass and aerobic power. That's encouraging because the workout is only four minutes of intense activity with periods of rest to make up the 20 minutes. This exercise can fit into anybody's schedule — even the most time-crunched individuals.

Strength training

There are other exercise routines you can add to have an all-round fitness plan. One of the best ways to prevent, and even reverse, bone and muscle loss is to add strength training into your exercise regime.

You do not need an expensive gym or weights and expensive machines. Lunges, squats, pushups, jump squats, pushing against a wall, and squatting against a wall are all examples of strength training. I recommend you do strength training twice a week. Your coordination, balance, and posture will improve, which can reduce your risk of falling by as much as 40 percent. This is crucial, especially as we get older. Studies have even shown strength training to be as effective as medication in decreasing arthritis pain.

Strength training can also help increase bone density and prevent fractures in most menopausal women. And for the millions of Americans with type 2 diabetes, strength training, along with a healthy diet, can help with glucose control. Strength training will boost your endorphins as well, which will make you feel great, sleep better, and help fight depression. Overall, strength training improves the quality of your life.

Aerobic exercises

Jogging, using an elliptical machine, and brisk walking are all examples of aerobic exercise. Aerobic exercises get your heart pumping more efficiently, improving the amount of oxygen in your blood and helping release endorphins, which act as natural painkillers and mood enhancers. Aerobic exercises also activate your immune system and increase your stamina over time.

Core exercises

The 29 core muscles located mostly in your back, abdomen, and pelvis provide the foundation for movement throughout your entire body. Strengthening them can help protect and support your back so that your spine and body will be less prone to injury. Core exercises also help you gain greater balance and stability.

Stretching

I love to stretch after a workout. My favorite is isolated stretching like callanetics, pilates, or yoga. These are different from the traditional type of stretching and an excellent way to get flexibility back into your core.

Summary

High-intensity interval training workouts like Peak Fitness play a vital role in promoting longevity and overall health.

Studies have shown that 12 weeks of high-intensity interval training not only can result in significant reductions in total abdominal, trunk, and visceral fat but can also give you significant increases in fat-free mass and aerobic power.

I recommend you do strength training twice a week. One of the best ways to prevent and even reverse bone and muscle loss, improve balance and flexibility, and improve your wellbeing is to add strength training twice a week into your regime.

It's imperative for you to listen to your body when you exercise. Start with a few intervals and then slowly increase your intensity as you go along. You should also learn how to adjust and set your fitness goals. By doing this, you will come up with a possible workout strategy that will provide you with the most effective and efficient benefits.

Chapter 14

Supplements

This is what I recommend as a basic regime for anybody over the age of 40.

Multivitamin

A good multivitamin should contain 1500mcg of vitamin A; 10 mcg of vitamin D; 100mcg of vitamin E; 250 mg of vitamin C; 25 mg each of B1, B2, B3, B5 and B6; 10 mcg of B12; 200 mcg of folic acid; and 50 mcg of biotin.

Multimineral

Your multimineral supplement should provide at least 150 mg of magnesium, 300 mg of calcium, 10 mg of zinc, 10 mg of iron, 2.5 mg of manganese, 25 mcg of selenium, 20 mcg of chromium, and some molybdenum, vanadium, and boron.

I find it easier to have a high potency multivitamin and mineral supplement 2 or 3 times daily to meet the required levels.

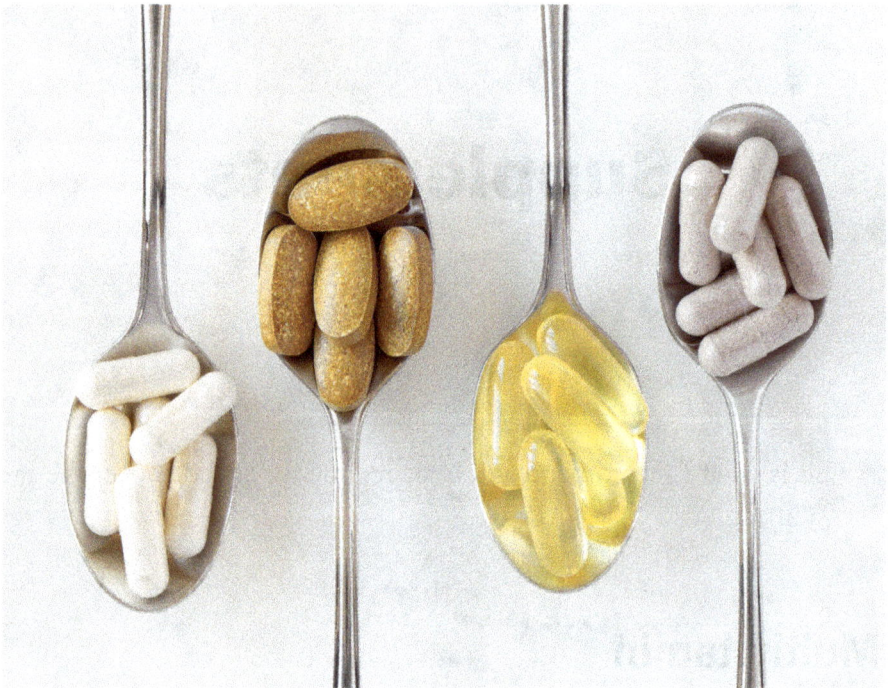

Vitamin C

It is well worth taking vitamin C separately because the amount you need will not fit into a multivitamin. The supplement should provide around 1,200 mg of Vitamin C.

Vitamin D

During the past decade, we have seen unprecedented research revealing the many beneficial roles vitamin D plays in keeping you healthy. It is a key player in your overall health. It turns on and off genes that can exacerbate or prevent many diseases.

One of the biggest problems facing today's high rates of chronic disease, besides poor diet and sedentary lifestyle, is an epidemic of vitamin D deficiency. It is estimated that 85 percent of Americans are deficient in vitamin D. A deficiency in Vitamin D increases individuals susceptibility to autoimmune conditions such as multiple sclerosis [MS], rheumatoid arthritis, type 1 diabetes, as well as some cancers and even dementia.

The most efficient way to increase your vitamin D levels is by exposing your skin to natural sunlight. Vitamin D from sunlight acts as a prohormone, converting rapidly through your skin. Whenever natural sun exposure is not an option, take a supplement of vitamin D3 15mcg daily. Over 70 years – 20mcg daily up to 125mcg daily if no exposure to sunlight is possible.

Vitamin K

Research continues to highlight the growing list of benefits that vitamin K does for your health. Vitamin K is probably where vitamin D was ten years ago on its appreciation as a vital nutrient that has far more advantages than originally thought.

Most people get enough K from their diet to maintain healthy blood clotting, but they don't get enough to offer protection against the health problems like dementia, prostate cancer, lung cancer, liver cancer, leukemia, osteoporosis, and infectious diseases such as pneumonia — and the list continues to grow.

Vitamin K exists in two basic forms: K1 and K2.

Vitamin K1

Found in green vegetables, K1 goes directly to your liver and helps you maintain a healthy blood clotting system. This is the kind of K that infants need to help prevent a severe bleeding disorder.

Vitamin K2

Bacteria produce this type of vitamin K. It is present in high quantities in your gut, but unfortunately, it is not absorbed from there and simply passes out in your stool. K2 goes straight to vessel walls, bones, and tissues other than your liver.

Who needs vitamin K?

If your family has a history of heart disease or osteoporosis, I strongly recommend you supplement vitamin K. Think of it as insurance to make sure your blood vessels don't clarify. If you don't eat many vegetables — especially spinach, kale, and green leafy vegetables — you will want to consider adding vitamin K to your supplement regime. Celiac disease, Crohn's disease, liver disease, and other conditions all interfere with nutrient absorption. Taking drugs such as cholesterol drugs, antibiotics, and aspirin will increase your risk of vitamin K deficiency.

The recommended dose is between 45 mcg and 185 mcg daily for adults. You must use caution on the higher doses if you take anticoagulants, but if you are generally healthy and not on these types of medications, 150 mcg daily is a good maintenance dose.

Who should not take vitamin K?

If you have experienced cardiac arrest or stroke or are prone to blood clotting, you should not take vitamin K without first consulting your doctor.

Amino Acids for Mind and Mood

Supplementing amino acids has been found to correct numerous mental health issues like depression, apathy, anxiousness, inability to relax, and poor memory and concentration. A good option is to supplement with a powder containing the right amount of free-forming amino acids. These don't require digestion the same way protein does, so they are easily absorbed into the body. A good powder should provide the following brain boosting amino acids:

Tryptophan	500 mg
Phenylalanine	1000 mg
GABA/taurine	1,500 mg
Glutamine/glutamic acid	2,000 mg

The protein powder can be mixed with yogurt, full cream milk as a shake, or with water.

Men should have three servings of protein-rich foods a day, and women should have two servings a day.

BCAA (branched chain amino acids)

These include the essential amino acids leucine, isoleucine, and valine. They are very popular among athletes, and there is some research validating their use. Numerous research studies have shown these three critical amino acids are paramount to consume, especially when you are dieting and exercising.

During exercise, your body uses a mix of glucose, fats, and even protein as a fuel source. When you diet and your carbohydrate intake is lower than normal, the percentage of protein your body uses for fuel (specifically leucine, isoleucine, and valine) dramatically increases. The body will pull those needed amino acids from the continuously circulating pool of amino acids in your bloodstream. And if not replenished from an outside source, your body will breakdown other areas of your body to supply this pool.

Studies have shown that subjects who consume an effective dose of BCAA's while dieting had greater levels of lean muscle mass retention than subjects who ingested a placebo. Results from one study concluded that the subjects consuming the high protein diet with branch chain amino acid supplements lost the greatest amount of body fat. Even more compelling is that the group supplementing with branch chain amino acids lost the greatest amount of fat from the abdominal and thigh regions, two areas of concern for many men and women in regards to fat loss. It is important to take doses of BCAA's before, during, and after exercise to maximize a workout program.

I recommend a free form BCAA with a ratio of 2:1:1 e.g. leucine 1100 mg, isoleucine 550 mg, and Valine 550 mg.

Summary

Vitamins play a major role in bodily functions, acting as coenzymes in chemical reactions. Vitamins support the nervous system, immune system, convert nutrients into energy, contribute to growth, aid in the clotting of blood, process protein, fats, and carbohydrates. Vitamin deficiencies can have serious consequences, such as mental disturbances, muscle weakness, anemia, disease, and infections.

Like Vitamins, minerals play a role in nearly every process your body performs. Minerals are not produced by the body, therefore need to be obtained from food or supplements. Minerals aid in proper growth and development, build and regulate cells. Their functions are enormously complex, and deficiencies can be very damaging such as muscle weakness, exhaustion, anemia, loss of cellular function to name a few.

I think anyone can benefit from a multivitamin and mineral which offers a wide variety of vitamins and minerals in one convenient capsule. This should cover all of the basis in addition to a nutritious diet.

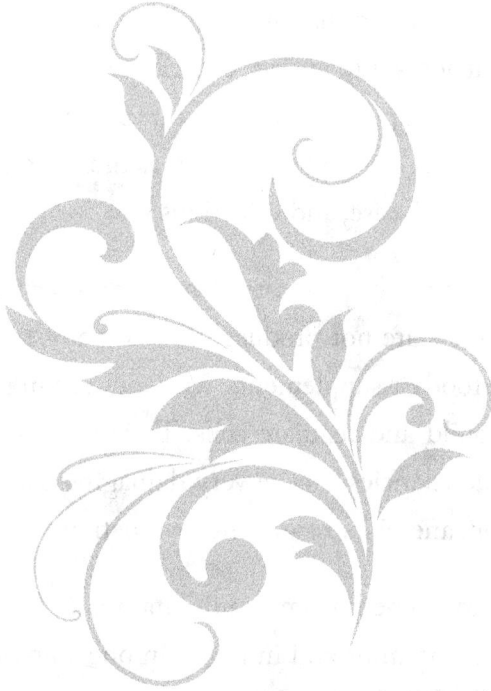

Chapter 15

Alzheimer's and Dementia Prevention and Memory-Boosting Supplements

Since nutrients are more potent in combination, my daily brain food that I take every day consists of supplementing a combination of the following mind and memory support nutrients. In combination with a basic exercise regime and a healthy diet, these supplements can help ward off Alzheimer's disease and dementia.

B Vitamins

The B vitamins could easily delay the onset of dementia or even eliminate it in combination with other prevention strategies. I recommend a homocysteine-lowering supplement. Reducing homocysteine with high-dose B vitamins really can halt the brain shrinkage associated with developing Alzheimer's. The results from Oxford University have been published online in the Public Library of Science.

	Prevention dose	Intervention dose
Thiamin [vitamin B1]	50mg	250mg
Niacin [vitamin B3]	100mg	500-1,000 mg
Pyridoxine Hydrochloride [B6]	50mg	100mg
Folic Acid	400mcg	1,200mcg
Cyanocobalmin [vitamin 12]	10mcg	100mcg
Pantothenic Acid [B5]	5mg	2,000 mg

Astaxanthin

A little-known carotenoid called astaxanthin is now believed to be the most beneficial antioxidant that nature offers. Astaxanthin' s benefits are numerous, promoting heart and eye health, UV-radiation protection, and improved athletic performance.

Astaxanthin is 550 times stronger than vitamin E and 6,000 times stronger than vitamin C! Astaxanthin has been proven to act on at least five different inflammation pathways and maintain balance within the system. Another significant advantage is the number of free radicals astaxanthin can handle at any given time. Most antioxidants, such as vitamins C, E, and others, can typically only handle one free radical at a time. But astaxanthin can handle multiple free radicals simultaneously — in some cases, more than 19 at the same time. When free radicals try to rob electrons from the astaxanthin molecule, they're just neutralized and absorbed into an electron cloud simultaneously.

Over the last few years, there have been at least 17 scientific studies on brain health showing that astaxanthin protects neurons and can slow the effects of age-related cognitive decline. Astaxanthin can cross the blood-brain barrier and the blood-retinal barrier, and it can provide antioxidant and anti-inflammatory protection to both the brain and the eyes.

Studies have also demonstrated that it improves blood flow and decreases blood pressure. It's very beneficial to your heart's mitochondrial membranes and can have a positive effect on blood chemistry, increasing HDL (the "healthy" cholesterol).

Astaxanthin will not work miracles overnight. It typically takes two weeks to one month to see the benefits. I take astaxanthin every day (5-10 mg per day), but you may receive benefit from as little as 4 mg per day. Those seeking to improve their heart health or athletic performance may want to take anywhere from 8-12 mg daily.

7-Keto-DHEA

This ingredient is a metabolite of DHEA (dehydroepiandrosterone), a natural hormone of the adrenal glands. Several studies show that this patented compound can have powerful fat burning effects in healthy individuals. People take 7-keto-DHEA to speed up the metabolism and heat production to promote weight loss. 7-keto-DHEA is also used to improve lean body mass and build muscle, increase the activity of the thyroid gland, boost the immune system, enhance memory, and slow aging.

A typical supplemental dosage of 7-keto-DHEA is 200-400 mg daily in two divided doses (100-200mg). Some limited evidence suggests that lower doses of 50-100 mg may also be beneficial.

DMAE

DMAE is probably the purest and most biologically available form of choline for purposes of oral supplementation. Choline boosts levels of the essential neurotransmitter acetylcholine.

While choline has difficulty crossing the blood-brain barrier, DMAE does not. It readily crosses the blood-brain barrier to increase acetylcholine biosynthesis in dosages of 25-200 mg daily. Studies show that by enhancing acetylcholine levels, IQ may be improved. DMAE may also help accurately control muscular force.

Phosphatidylserine (PS)

As mentioned in a previous chapter, Phosphatidylserine is a naturally occurring phospholipid found in the body. Phospholipids are important constituents of cell membranes with extensive functions in the human body. PS has been reported to be useful for cognitive improvement and recovery in sports and physical training. More specifically, PS is thought to have positive effects on mental function and mood. There have been several studies on patients with Alzheimer's which suggest they experienced improved mood and response times when taking PS.

The other benefits of PS use are associated with physical activity, as it has shown to promote a positive hormone balance. Improved recovery time, coupled with reduced fatigue and muscle soreness (DOMS), has been reported after exercise while using PS. Furthermore, it is thought to exhibit anti-stress properties by decreasing elevated levels of cortisol post-training.

Cortisol is a hormone known for muscle breakdown and catabolism and is also associated with weight gain if elevated for prolonged periods of time. I recommend 300 mg as a dietary supplement. For the treatment of Alzheimer's disease and other age-related memory impairment, I recommend a dose of 100 mg of phosphatidylserine taken three times daily.

Carnitine

Carnitine is a compound that is biosynthesized from the essential amino acids methionine and lysine. However, when carnitine undergoes the process of acetylation, which involves adding an acetyl group to a molecule, it has a significantly improved ability to cross the blood-brain barrier. This enhances the effectiveness of L-carnitine per dose, allowing it to reach the brain more quickly, and this is what makes acetyl-L-carnitine a more efficient product. This is the same as the relationship between choline and acetylcholine, which, as you know, is an essential neurotransmitter in the brain.

The effects of supplementation have been widely researched in various areas, including anti-aging, mental and sports performance, anxiety and mood improvement, weight loss, and treatment of diseases such as Alzheimer's and Parkinson's. It's a great antioxidant, as it has been shown to prevent spatial memory impairment in studies.

Spatial memory is the part of the memory that is responsible for recording the environment and one's spatial awareness to it. Spatial memory is required for finding one's way around a city or a familiar location, for example. These are often referred to as your "cognitive maps" and are represented in working short and long-term memory. Furthermore,

Carnitine has been shown to have a vital role in maintaining healthy brain function, memory, and mood as we age. Carnitine improves cognition in the brain, significantly reversed age-associated decline in the mitochondrial membrane.

Finally, carnitine is also vital for the transport of fatty acids during the process of creating metabolic energy. In other words, it facilitates the process of breaking down fat stores for energy, and so it can be helpful during exercise and dieting. As a dietary supplement, take one scoop (500 mg) one to three times per day.

Black Seed Oil: A True Panacea

There have been over 600 scientific peer-reviewed articles published about the benefits of black seed oil, and one thing is clear: the healing prowess of black seed oil is astonishing, and it is unbelievable that most people haven't heard of it.

Black seed oil is a real panacea, able to help cure everything from allergies to hypertension.

The liver is one of the most important organs in the body. Every toxin gets processed through the liver to keep your mind and body healthy and happy. for those who have struggled with poor liver function due to alcohol consumption or medication side effects, black seed oil could significantly speed the healing process. In recent studies, scientists discovered that black seed oil benefits the function of the liver and helps prevent both damage and disease.

Black seed oil improves glucose tolerance as efficiently as metformin; yet has not shown significant adverse effects. This is huge because metformin, one of the most commonly prescribed type 2 diabetes drugs, can have dozens of side effects, including constipation, bloating, gas, indigestion, heartburn, flushing of the skin, headache, metallic taste in the mouth, stomach pain, muscle pain and weight loss. There are few natural remedies on the planet that have the healing powers similar.

The Journal of Diabetes and Metabolic Disorders published a study systemically reviewing the literature for plants that have anti-obesity properties, was amongst the most efficient natural remedies on the planet. Not traditionally believed to treat obesity, black seed oil is a remarkable anti-inflammatory agent that is known to help people lose weight in the same way that it helps people with diabetes. Black seed oil has helped millions shed excess weight, control appetite, and improve, blood glucose levels, cholesterol, triglycerides, and glucose absorption in the intestine.

A unique black seed oil benefit is its powerful antioxidant and antimicrobial properties that help restore hair loss by strengthening hair follicles and promotes the strengthening of the hair roots.

Black seed oil benefits on the skin and other cells are profoundly healing. Black seed oil was found as effective as the skin cream Betamethasone in improving the quality of life and decreasing the severity of hand eczema. When you consider that black seed oil has virtually no side effects, the benefits far exceed medical intervention!

With all these health benefits, I recommend everybody has black seed oil in their medicine cabinets. As a supplement for adults, take 1/2 a teaspoon gradually increasing over a few days to 1 to 2 teaspoons daily (with a small amount of food or drink) and gradually increase over few days.

Chapter 16

Smoking

Smoking depletes the body and the brain of essential vitamins and minerals. Supplementing may be the most important thing you can do for yourself in the fight against toxic free radicals. Smoking is very dangerous for your health, and it goes without saying that the best way to prevent free radical damage is to quit. But easier said than done; if you cannot, you need to protect yourself the best you can by supplementing these vitamins and minerals that are depleted.

An estimated 42.1 million adults in the United States are cigarette smokers. Smoking causes 40,000 deaths per year in the country — which is a staggering 1,300 deaths per day.

Antioxidants such as vitamins C and E can prevent this damage. In fact, one of the most important functions in the body is that of an antioxidant, and it is vitally important to smoking and vitamin depletion.

Smokers will break down vitamin C as well as several of the B vitamins that are essential for cell and organ oxidation almost fifty percent faster than non-smokers. Vitamin C is imperative in our cellular fluids and collagen production, and it helps vitamin E in retaining its active form of fighting the growth of free radicals. Vitamin E is the most effective antioxidant in breaking the free dramatic change.

Collagen, which is a protein constituent of connective tissue, bone, and tendons, helps in preventing wrinkles and sallow skin conditions. The oxidation process of Vitamin E is also imperative to smokers.

Vitamin B6 is also depleted by smoking and is instrumental in turning proteins and carbohydrates into the form of energy.

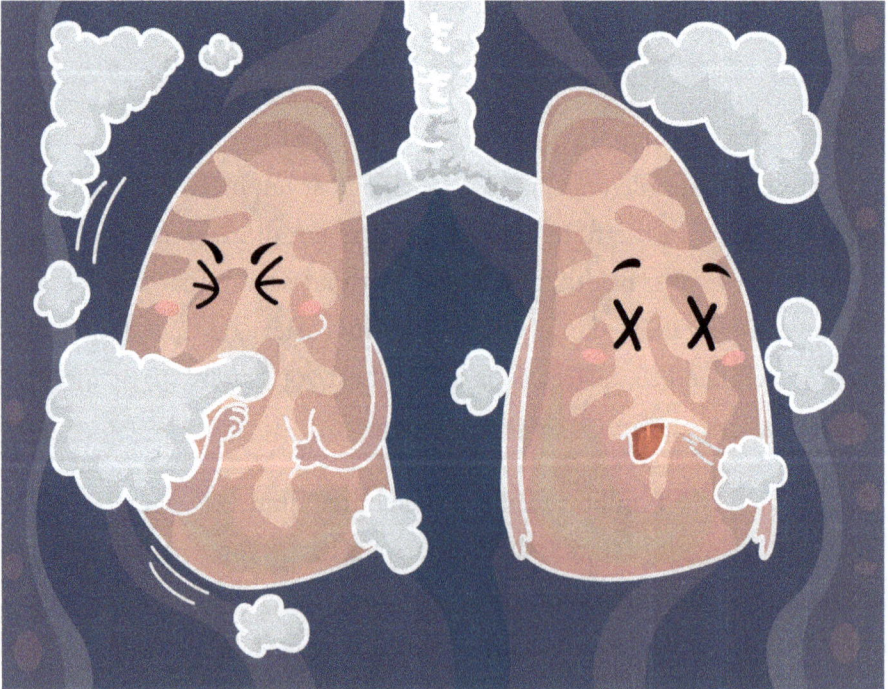

If you smoke, the only sensible way to avoid smoking-related diseases is to give up. However, as I have already said, easier said than done. In the meantime, the following nutrients are necessary for preserving your health and minimizing damage.

A multivitamin/mineral that contains all the essential vitamins and minerals.

- Beta-carotene 15mg – 30mg per day
- Vitamin B-complex supplement containing:
- Biotin 300 mcg
- Folic acid 400 mcg
- Vitamin B3 (niacin) 20 mg
- Vitamin B5 (pantothenic acid) 10 mg
- Vitamin B2 (riboflavin) 1.7 mg
- Vitamin B1 (thiamine) 1.5 mg
- Vitamin B6 (pyridoxine) 2 mg
- Vitamin B12 (cobalamin) 6 mcg
- Calcium 1,500 mg
- Vitamin C 180 to 2,000 mg
- Vitamin E 20 mg daily

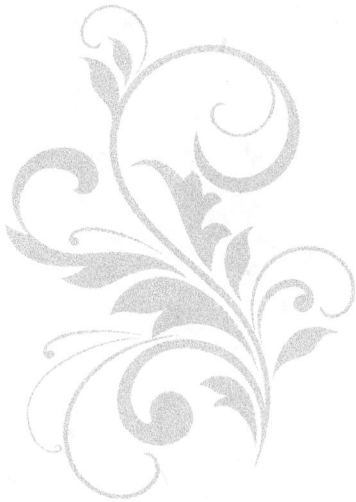

Conclusion

That's it - the end of this book is just the beginning of a brand new you. You have wanted to lose weight, get fit, healthy, vibrant, motivated, and live a long happy life and you deserve it. You succeed because of the choices you make. Choices equal destiny. Every time you choose a meal, food, snack or drink, you are making a decision that affects you and your body in a positive or a negative way. Dump the junk. What matters now is that you continue to build a life for yourself free from debilitating health issues, mental health issues and prescription drugs.

Here's to your new life.

I have added a few recipes in the next section to help you navigate the ketogenic diet.

Recipes for the Ketogenic Diet

H ere are some examples to help you work with the ketogenic diet described earlier in the book.

Examples

Breakfast

- Two eggs, fried in butter or olive oil
- 1 ounce of chopped onion, or another low carb vegetable
- 1 ounce of cheese
- Four slices bacon

- Coffee with 1 ounce heavy cream

OR

- Protein shake made with chocolate whey protein powder
- 16 ounces unsweetened almond milk
- 2 ounces heavy cream

Lunch

- 6 ounces baked fish with dill butter sauce
- 1 cup cauliflower, chopped and sautéed in olive oil or butter
- 1 cup of salad sprinkled with blue cheese and dressed with a tablespoon of full-fat mayonnaise
- Water or unsweetened flavored sparkling water

OR

- 3 cups of salad greens
- 6 ounces of chicken breast strips, cooked in butter or olive oil
- 4 teaspoons of high fat, low carb salad dressing
- 1 ounce of full-fat cheese
- One celery stalk with 1 ounce of cream cheese
- Water or unsweetened flavored sparkling water

OR

- 4 ounces of prime mince, mixed with two chopped onions and spices, patted into patties
- A handful of low GI vegetables, fried in olive oil or butter
- Cauliflower cheese made with full-fat cheese
- Coffee with double cream

OR

- 6 ounces of smoked ham
- 1 cup sliced summer squash, sautéed in butter or olive oil
- 1 ounce of parmesan cheese, sprinkled over squash
- One or two celery stalks stuffed with a mixture of blue cheese and cream cheese
- Sparkling water, still water, tea, or coffee

Dinner

- 6 ounces of grilled or pan fried steak
- Mushrooms sautéed in butter
- Broccoli or other low carb vegetables
- Water, unsweetened flavored sparkling water, or other unsweetened beverage
- Coffee with heavy cream

<u>OR</u>

- 6 ounces of pork chop baked in a garlic cream
- 2 cups shredded cabbage sautéed in butter with salad greens with high-fat dressing
- Water, unsweetened flavored sparkling water, or other unsweetened beverage
- Coffee with heavy cream

<u>OR</u>

- 6 ounces of salmon topped with parmesan cream sauce and baked
- 2 cups spinach sautéed with onions and garlic
- Salad greens with high-fat dressing
- Water or unsweetened flavored sparkling water
- Coffee with heavy cream if it doesn't affect sleep or tea

Recipes

Easy egg salad

A delicious, simple, but tasty, egg salad recipe.
Serves: 4 servings

Ingredients:

- 6 eggs
- 2 tablespoons mayonnaise
- 1 teaspoon of Dijon mustard
- 1 teaspoon of lemon juice
- 1/4 teaspoon of lite salt (for potassium)
- Kosher salt and pepper to taste

Instructions:

Place the eggs in a small to medium saucepan. Cover eggs with about an inch of cold water. Bring it to a boil for ten minutes or until eggs are hard. Remove from heat and cool. Peel the eggs. I place them under cold running water if they are still too hot.

Add the eggs to a food processor and chop. Stir in the mustard, mayonnaise, lemon juice and salt and pepper. Taste and adjust as necessary. I love this served with crispy lettuce leaves and bacon for wrapping if desired. (Optional)

Approximate nutrition info per serving: 166 calories, 14g fat, 85 g net carbs, 10 g protein Serving size: 1/3 cup

Meat Bagel

Ingredients

- 1-1/2 onions, finely diced
- 1 tablespoon of butter/grass fed ghee/bacon fat etc.
- 2 pounds of ground pork
- Two large eggs
- 2/3 cup tomato sauce
- One teaspoon of paprika
- One teaspoon of salt
- 1/2 teaspoon of pepper

Instructions

1. Preheat the oven to 400 degrees. Line a baking dish with parchment paper.
2. Sauté the onions over medium heat with some cooking fat like butter, grass fed ghee, etc. Sauté for about 10 minutes until cooked but not brown. Allow the onions to cool before adding them to the meat.
3. In a bowl, mix all of the ingredients including the cooked onions. Mix well to evenly distribute the spices.
4. Divide the meat into six portions. Using your hands, roll one patty into a ball and then push a whole in the middle, and slightly flatten to form the appearance of a bagel.
5. Place the bagel looking meat in the dish and repeat with each of the portions of meat.
6. Bake for 40 minutes or until the patty is fully cooked.
7. Allow the meat bagels to cool. Slice the patty bagel just like a regular bagel. Fill the patty bagel with the topping such as tomato slices, lettuce, onions, etc. This is delicious

Zucchini Chips with Smoked Paprika

2 servings

Ingredients

- 1 medium zucchini
- 1/2 teaspoon of salt
- 2 teaspoons of olive oil
- 1 teaspoon smoked paprika
- 1/4 teaspoon of ground pepper

Instructions

1. Slice zucchini crosswise into 1/4 inch thick slices using a mandolin slicer or a sharp knife.
2. Place the sliced zucchini in layers into a colander or sieve, sprinkling with a little salt with each layer. Let drain one hour.
3. Preheat oven to 250 F and oil parchment paper and line a baking sheet with oiled parchment paper.
4. Wrap zucchini slices into a paper towel for a thorough drying and place on prepared baking sheet. Brush tops with remaining oil and sprinkled with paprika and ground pepper.
5. Bake for about 45 minutes and let the chips stay inside turned off oven until crispy for about 1 hour. Enjoy!

Zucchini Fritters

Ingredients

- 4-5 medium zucchini squash (courgettes)
- 1/2 cup flour
- 1/4 cup chopped mint
- 3.5 ounces of feta, crumbled
- 2 free-range eggs, lightly whisked
- Freshly ground black pepper

Instructions

These are such a good snack or alongside steak or meatballs.
They go great with a sauce of natural yogurt, chopped garlic, sea salt, and chopped mint.

Grate zucchini and place in a colander, sprinkle with 1/2 teaspoon sea salt and leave to drain for 30 minutes. Press to remove any excess liquid with paper towel and place in a bowl along with mint, crumbled feta and flour. Make a well in the center and add eggs, mix until combined. Season to taste with freshly ground black pepper. Heat a film of oil in a frying pan over medium heat, place spoonfuls of batter into the pan and cook fritters until golden on both sides. Remove from the pan and drain on paper towels.

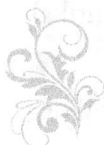

Ricotta Meatball Recipe

Ingredients

- 4 ounces of white onion, minced
- 1 tablespoon butter
- 1 cup cold whole milk ricotta cheese
- 1 large egg
- 1 and 1/2 teaspoons of sea salt
- 1/2 teaspoon of ground black pepper
- A pinch of herbs of your choice
- 4 ounces of dry, hard cheese
- 1 pound of ground beef

Instructions

1. Preheat oven to 350 degrees.
2. Sauté onions in butter until translucent, then remove from heat and cool for 10 minutes.
3. Chop the hard cheese while onions are cooling and then mince the cheese in a food processor until crumbly. Set aside.
4. Combine ricotta cheese and egg in a mixing bowl. Whisk until smooth.
5. Add the salt, pepper, and spices and mix.
6. Add onions and minced hard cheese. Mix well.
7. Add the beef and mix until all ingredients are combined.
8. Roll mix into balls.
9. Bake the meatballs at 350 degrees until cooked through and browned about 20 minutes.

Asian Cabbage Stir-Fry

Ingredients

- 1.5 pounds of green cabbage
- 5.2 ounces of butter
- 1.3 pounds of ground beef, lamb chicken or pork
- 1 teaspoon salt
- 1 teaspoon onion powder
- 1/4 teaspoon ground black pepper
- 1 tablespoon white wine vinegar
- Three spring onions, in slices
- 1 teaspoon chili flakes
- 1 tablespoon finely chopped fresh ginger
- 1 tablespoon sesame oil
- 1 cup mayonnaise
- 1 tablespoon wasabi paste

Instructions

1. Shred the cabbage finely with a food processor or with a knife
2. Place 3 ounces of butter in a large frying on medium high. Fry the cabbage until it softens but not browned. It takes a while.
3. Add the vinegar and spices. Fry and stir for a few minutes more. Put the cabbage in a bowl.
4. Melt the rest of the butter in the same frying pan. Add garlic, chili flakes, and ginger and sauté for a few minutes.
5. Add ground meat and brown until the meat is thoroughly cooked and most of the juices have evaporated. Lower the heat a little.
6. Add spring onions and cabbage. Stir until everything is hot. Salt and pepper to taste.
7. Mix the mayonnaise and wasabi paste. Start with ½ tablespoon and add more until you think it tastes good.
8. Add the sesame oil before serving.

Baked Salmon with Lemon and Butter

Ingredients

- 1 tablespoon olive oil
- 3.3 pounds salmon
- 1 teaspoon sea salt
- Ground black pepper
- 7 ounces of butter
- 1 lemon

Instructions

1. Preheat the oven to 390 degrees.
2. Pour olive oil into a baking dish. Place the salmon with the skin down and add a generous amount of salt and pepper
3. Thinly slice the lemon and place on top of the salmon. Cover with half of the butter in thin slabs
4. Bake on the middle rack for about 20 to 30 minutes, depending on size.
5. Melt the butter in a small pan until it starts to bubble, then remove from heat and let it cool a little and add some lemon juice.
6. Serve the fish with the lemon butter and a side dish of your choice. See below for suggestions.

Chicken Breast with Herb Butter

Ingredients

- 4 chicken breasts
- 2 tablespoons butter
- 5.5 ounces herb butter
- Salt and pepper to taste

Instructions

1. Spoon a generous amount of butter into a pan (flavored is even better, such as herb butter, garlic butter or bacon butter).
2. Fry the chicken in olive oil or butter on medium heat until the fillets are browned and well-done.
3. Add the salt and pepper to taste. Turn the temperature down towards the end to avoid drying the chicken meat.
4. Serve the chicken and herb butter with a tasty salad or with cauliflower mash or a side dish of your choice.

Scrambled Eggs

The great thing about scrambled eggs is that the butter is blended in with the eggs. For a more decadent meal, you can add cream to the mix! Scrambled eggs are the perfect breakfast.

- 3 eggs
- Four tablespoons butter
- Salt and pepper

Instructions

1. Beat the eggs together with some salt and pepper using a fork.
2. Let the butter melt carefully in a pan over medium heat. The butter should not turn brown!
3. Pour the eggs into the pan and stir for 1 to 2 minutes until they turn creamy. Remember that the eggs are still cooking even after you've put them on your plate.
4. Have your scrambled eggs together with different side dishes, such as salmon, avocado, bacon, deli meat, sausages, cheese, fresh mozzarella, and feta cheese.

Mushroom Omelet

This is perfect for a ketosis breakfast.

Ingredients

- 3 eggs
- Butter, for frying
- 1 ounce shredded cheese
- 1 onion
- 2 to 3 mushrooms
- Salt and pepper

Instructions

1. Whisk the eggs into a batter with a fork. Add the salt, pepper, and spices.
2. Melt butter in a frying pan and pour in the batter when the butter has melted.
3. When the omelet looks firm but still has a little raw egg on top, sprinkle mushrooms, cheese, and onion on top (optional).
4. When the eggs start to turn golden brown, ease the edges of the omelet and fold it over in half. Remove the frying pan from the heat and slide the omelet onto a plate.
5. Serve the omelet with a crispy salad or just on its own.

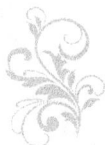

Low-Carb Cauliflower Mash

This is a classic, versatile side dish that goes great with just about anything.

Ingredients

- 1 pound of cauliflower
- 3.5 ounces grated parmesan cheese
- 3.5 ounces butter
- 1/2 lemon, juice, and zest
- Olive oil (optional)

Instructions

1. Cut the cauliflower into florets.
2. Steam the cauliflower in plenty of lightly salted water for about 5 minutes — just enough to retain a somewhat firm texture.
3. In a food processor, hand blender, or with a potato masher blend all other ingredients.

Broccoli and Cauliflower in Cheese

This is a delicious substitute for potatoes or rice on a ketogenic diet. Here's a vegetable dish that goes great with all kinds of meat, but also as a main dish.

Ingredients

- 8 ounces cauliflower
- 1 pound broccoli, chopped
- 5.2 ounces shredded cheese
- 1.5 ounces butter
- Four tablespoons sour cream
- 1/2 cup fresh oregano or fresh thyme
- Salt and pepper

Instructions

1. Chop the veggies and fry in butter.
2. Add the cheese and sour cream and stir. Season.
3. Serve with fried chicken breast, fried in butter until golden brown and fully cooked through.

Ground Beef with Red Peppers

Ingredients:

- Onions
- Coconut Oil
- Ground Beef
- Spinach
- Spices
- Red Pepper

Instructions:

1. Dice an onion.
2. Put coconut oil in the pan, add onion, and stir for a couple of minutes
3. Add ground beef.
4. Add some spices (I use a spice mix, but salt and pepper work fine).
5. Add spinach.
6. If you want to spice things up a bit, add some black pepper and chili powder.
7. Fry in a wok or stir-fry until ready, serve with a sliced bell pepper.

Cheeseburgers Without the Bun

I love this simple, easy meal. Burgers without the bun, but with flavor and delicious cheeses, served with lettuce.

Ingredients:

- Butter
- Hamburger patties
- Cheddar Cheese
- Cream Cheese
- Salsa
- Spices
- Spinach

Instructions:

1. Put butter in a pan.
2. Fry meat patties that have had spices added.
3. Turn until close to being ready.
4. Add cream cheese and a few slices of cheddar cheese on top.
5. Turn down the heat and put a lid on the pan until the cheese melts.
6. Serve with some lettuce for the crunch. To make burgers even, juicier add some salsa on top.

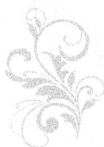

Fried Chicken Breast Pieces

I don't always eat chicken breasts — I find them too dry — but adding lots of butter makes them much more palatable.

Ingredients:

- Chicken Breast
- Butter
- Salt and Pepper
- Curry powder
- Garlic
- Vegetables

Instructions:

1. Cut chicken breast into small pieces.
2. Add butter to the frying pan and add the chicken pieces.
3. Add a bunch of salt, pepper, curry, and garlic powder.
4. Stir fry in a wok until the chicken gets a brown, crunchy texture.
5. Serve with some greens or broccoli.

One-Pan Baked Chicken Thighs

Servings: 4
Prep Time: 15 minutes
Cook Time: 30 minutes

Ingredients

- Four chicken thighs (deboned, skin on)
- Two zucchinis, 1/2 cup carrot (sliced)
- 1 cup daikon radish
- 1/4 cup olive oil
- 2 tablespoon balsamic vinegar
- 1-inch cube minced ginger

Instructions

1. Preheat oven to 350 degrees F. Pat boneless chicken thighs dry with handy towel or paper towel.
2. Place the chicken thighs with skin on a baking dish greased with butter.
3. Chop the vegetables and put them around the chicken.
4. Whisk together your sauce ingredients (olive oil, balsamic vinegar, and ginger) and pour over your chicken and veggies. Season with salt and pepper and bake for 30 minutes. For extra crispiness, grill for about 3 to 5 minutes (keep an eye on it! All ovens are different!). Enjoy with cauliflower mash.

References

1) Protein in nutrition. (2015, March 02). Retrieved March 07, 2015, from **https://en.wikipedia.org/wiki/Protein_in_nutrition**

2) Omega-6 Oil. (n.d.). Retrieved March 10, 2015, from **http://omega6.wellwise.org/**

3) Saturated and Trans fats | The Heart Foundation. (n.d.). **https://heartfoundation.org.au/healthy-eating/ food-and-nutrition/fats-and-cholesterol/ saturated-and-trans-fat**

4) Gavin, M. L. (Ed.). (2013, July).
What's Cholesterol? Retrieved January 14, 2014,
from **http://kidshealth.org/en/kids/cholesterol.html**

5) Health Benefits. (n.d.). Retrieved June 07, 2015,
from **https://www.organicfacts.net/health-benefits**

6) **https://authoritynutrition.com/
how-much-water-should-you-drink-per-day/**

7) **http://www.mayoclinic.org/healthy-lifestyle/
nutrition-and-healthy-eating/in-depth/fat/art-20045550**

8) Water: How much should you drink every day? (n.d.).
Retrieved January 20, 2017, from **http://beautywellnessnews.
arbonne.com/articles/water-how-much-should-you-drink-
every-day.shtml**

9) Glycemic Index. (n.d.). Retrieved August 08, 2011,
from http://www.glycemicindex.com/

10) The Failure of Low-Calorie Diets | Official website of the
Montignac Method. (n.d.). **http://montignac.com/en/
the-failure-of-low-calorie-diets/**

11) **http://articles.mercola.com/sites/articles/archive/2007/08/23/
is-sugar-more-addictive-than-cocaine.aspx**

12) M, K. (n.d.). Cilantro Lime Rice. Retrieved January 10, 2017,
from **http://www.thegardengrazer.com/2013/05/cilantro-lime-
rice.html**

13) (2013, August 16). White Rice Nutrition Facts. Retrieved July 01, 2016, from **http://www.livestrong.com/ article/258776-white-rice-nutrition-facts**

14) **http://healthyeating.sfgate.com/potatoes-turn-sugar-digested-4400.html**

15) Zorn, M., Gazdecki, A., & Lombardo, C. (2014, July 03). Who Invented High Fructose Corn Syrup? Retrieved March 10, 2015, from **http://visionlaunch.com/who-invented-high-fructose-corn-syrup/**]

16) **http://www.ketogenic-diet-resource.com/low-carb-dieting.html**

17) Why Is Intermittent Fasting Highly Recommended? (n.d.). Retrieved August 28, 2014, from **http://fitness.mercola. com/sites/fitness/archive/2013/01/18/intermittent-fasting-approach.aspx**

18) What the Science Says About Intermittent Fasting. (2013). Retrieved November 21, 2014, from **http://healthimpactnews. com/2013/what-the-science-says-about-intermittent-fasting/**

19) Obesity data and stats. (n.d.). Retrieved November 24, 2016, from **http://www.health.govt.nz/nz-health-statistics/ health-statistics-and-data-sets/obesity-data-and-stats**

20) **http://www.radionz.co.nz/news/world/300879/ world-faces-%27unrelenting-march%27-of-diabetes**

21) Obesity / Weight Loss / Fitness Today. (n.d.). Retrieved March News from Medical News 10, 2017

22) Ketogenic Diet Resource. (n.d.). Retrieved March 11, 2016, from **http://www.ketogenic-diet-resource.com/**

23) Jr., R. E., Psy.D., S. S., Ph.D., L. G., & Ph.D., S. W. (n.d.). Retrieved May 14, 2015, from **https://www.psychologytoday. com/basics/dopamine**

24) Brain.co.uk. (n.d.). Retrieved March 11, 2017, from **http://www.brain.co.uk/**

25) **http://www.vipdispensary.com/product/ Essential_Therapeutics_Brain_Fog_Formula_60/ htc_chronic_fatigue_fibromyalgia**

26) **https://www.patrickholford.com/advice/ natural-mind-memory-enhancers**

27) **http://www.helpguide.org/articles/sleep/cant-sleep-insomnia-treatment.htm**

28) 5-Hydroxytryptophan (5-HTP). (n.d.). Retrieved March 11, 2017, from **https://umm.edu/health/medical/altmed/ supplement/5hydroxytryptophan-5htp**

29) 2012 Archive. (n.d.). Retrieved July 11, 2014, from **http://www. hypoglycemia.asn.au/2012**

30) **http://articles.mercola.com/sites/articles/archive/2008/08/14/ is-krill-oil-48-times-better-than-fish-oil.aspx**

31) Purdy, M. C. (2016, January 25). Sleep loss precedes Alzheimer's symptoms | The Source | Washington University in St. Louis. Retrieved March 11, 2016, from **https://source.wustl. edu/2013/03/sleep-loss-precedes-alzheimer-symptoms/**

32) K. (n.d.). Seven hours of sleep is just about optimal. Retrieved March 11, 2016, from **http://www.motherjones.com/ kevin-drum/2014/07/seven-hours-sleep-just-about-optimal**

33) How Sleep Works. (n.d.). Retrieved March 11, 2017, from **https://sleepfoundation.org/how-sleep-works**

34) Understanding the stress response - palousemindfulness.com. (n.d.). Retrieved March 11, 2017, from **https://www.bing.com/cr? IG=1929F64A65A04F12A14927B4C54286CC&CID=3A6681 FFF1326D07073E8BBDF0036CCC&rd=1&h=8Zcw429D8X lNdqN8g5HyG7DRxtjt3ymYgyPhXUnceBM&v=1&r=https% 3a%2f%2fpalousemindfulness.com%2fdocs%2funderstanding-stress.pdf&p=DevEx,5039.1**

35) **https://adrenalfatiguesolution.com/ what-are-the-adrenal-glands/**

36) Adrenal Fatigue Treatment - 15 Essential Recovery Tips. (2015, August 26). Retrieved March 11, 2016, from **http://naturalsociety.com/ adrenal-fatigue-treatment-15-essential-rescue-recovery-tips/**

37) P. (2009, January 06). Reduce your risk of heart disease. Retrieved March 11, 2014, from **https://www.patrickholford.com/advice/ reduce-your-risk-of-heart-disease**

38) InfoPOEMs. (2008, November 06). Retrieved January 14, 2014, from **http://onlinelibrary.wiley.com/doi/10.1002/dat.20449/full**

39) What Is Ablation of Atrial Fibrillation? (n.d.). Retrieved March 11, 2017, from **http://www.healthline.com/health/heart-disease**

40) /Heart-Attack-Symptoms-in-Women_UCM_436448_Article.jspv Heart Attack Symptoms in Women. (n.d.). Retrieved March 11, 2017, from **http://www.heart.org/HEARTORG/Conditions/ HeartAttack/WarningSignsofaHeartAttack**

41) Risk | Look for Heart Attack Symptoms and Signs. (n.d.). Retrieved March 07, 2015, from **https://herheart.org.au/risk/ signs-and-symptoms-of-heart-attack/**

42) Alzheimer's disease and Sleep. (n.d.). Retrieved March 11, 2017, from **https://sleepfoundation.org/sleep-disorders-problems/ alzheimers-disease-and-sleep**

43) Shackford, B. (n.d.). Vitamin C halts aggressive colorectal cancer: study | Cornell Chronicle. Retrieved March 11, 2017

44) Extra Happiness. (n.d.). Retrieved March 11, 2017, from **http://extrahappiness.com/happiness/**

45) **http://articles.mercola.com/peak-fitness.aspx**

46) (n.d.). Anti-Aging | Telemeres To Change The Human Aging Process. Retrieved March 13, 2013, from **http://articles.mercola. com/sites/articles/archive/2010/02/23/science-finally-reveals- how-you-can-actually-revese-aging.aspx**

47) **http://articles.mercola.com/peak-fitness.aspx**

48) **https://www.patrickholford.com/advice/ which-health-supplements-to-take**

49) The Delicate Dance Between Vitamins D and K. (n.d.). Retrieved March 11, 2014, from **http://articles.mercola.com/**

sites/articles/archive/2011/03/26/the-delicate-dance-between-vitamins-d-and-k.aspx#!

50) The Delicate Dance between Vitamins D and K. (n.d.). Retrieved March 11, 2014, from **http://articles.mercola.com/ sites/articles/archive/2011/03/26/the-delicate-dance-between-vitamins-d-and-k.aspx#!**

51) ProLineSportsNutrition.com - Amino Acids BCAA. (n.d.). Retrieved March 11, 2017, from **http://www.bing.com/cr? IG=332AADE79240466D8C2104F082C210D4&CID= 21D598A203CE6421203692E002FF65C8&rd=1&h=e-9FqFIgyLhwVcgKsWssj_F3OOsuxj8Pbb9RCWtdDbs &v=1&r=http%3a%2f%2fwww.prolinesportsnutrition. com%2famino-acids-bcaa%3fb%3d1&p=DevEx,5059.**

52) Vitamins and Supplements. (n.d.). Retrieved March 11, 2017, from **http://www.livestrong.com/sscat/vitamins-supplements/v**

53) Astaxanthin: High-Quality Antioxidant Supplement. (n.d.). Retrieved March 11, 2016, from **http://products.mercola.com/ astaxanthin**

54) **https://examine.com/supplements/7-keto-dhea/**

55) **http://www.mindnutrition.com/products/phosphatidylserine**

56) **https://store.mindnutrition.com/ nootropics/21-acetyl-l-carnitine**

57) **https://draxe.com/black-seed-oil-benefits/**

58) Smoking and Vitamin Loss. (n.d.). Retrieved February 21, 2016, from **http://www.humanvitaminhealth.com/smokingandvitaminloss.html**

59) Diabetes. (n.d.). Retrieved November 21, 2016, from **http://www.who.int/mediacentre/factsheets/fs312/en/**

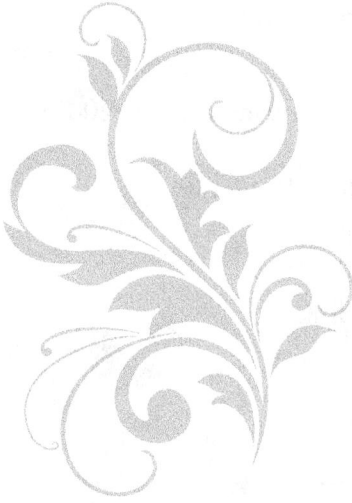

Recommended Books

Parker S. *The Concise Human Body Book*.
London: Dorling Kindersley; 2009.

Montignac, M. (2001). *Eat well stay young*.
Montignac Publishing.

Hofmekler O, Holtzberg D. *The Warrior Diet*.
Figline Valdarno: Ciccarelli; 2005.

Atkins RC. *Dr. Atkins New Diet Revolution*.
New York: M. Evans and Co; 1992.

Willett W, Skerrett PJ, Giovannucci EL, Callahan M.
Eat, Drink, and Be Healthy: the Harvard Medical School Guide to Healthy Eating. New York: Simon & Schuster Source; 2001.

Mansfield J. *The Six Secrets of Successful Weight Loss.*
London: Hammersmith Health; 2012.

Miller JB, Colagiuri S, Foster-Powell K.
The New Glucose Revolution: Losing Weight.
Sydney: Hodder Headline; 2003.

Holford P. *The New Optimum Nutrition Bible.*
Berkeley, CA: Crossing Press; 2005.

Greenfield, S. (1997). *The human brain: A guided tour.*
New York: Basic Books.

Holford, P. (2003). *Optimum nutrition for the mind.*
London: Piatkus.

Montignac, M. (2010).
The French GI diet for women: 100 low carb recipes.
Monaco: Alpen Editions.

Index

A

Alzheimer's 8, 9, 12-14, 22, 34, 50, 60, 85, 88, 103, 123-131, 149, 150, 152, 153, 186, 188

Amino Acids 7, 9, 18-20, 33, 37, 81-83, 89, 91, 145, 146, 153, 189

B

Blood pressure , 12, 15, 23, 25, 39, 45, 52, 88, 102, 105, 107, 108, 110, 111, 117-119, 121, 127, 130, 151

C

Calories 6, 27, 29, 37, 49, 50, 54, 56, 60, 75, 76, 166

Carbohydrates 6, 12, 18, 29-31, 33, 34, 42, 50, 54, 58, 75, 81, 108, 125, 147, 158

Cholesterol

Cholesterol 5, 8, 15, 22-27, 39, 45, 110, 116-119, 121, 127, 133, 144, 151, 155, 184

Coconut oil 5, 25, 26, 51, 52, 58, 60, 97, 99, 111, 112, 114, 178

D

Dementia 8, 9, 13, 14, 91, 123-125, 143, 149, 150

F

Fasting 6, 15, 54-62, 185

Fatigue 8, 22, 34, 81, 89, 91, 94, 101, 108, 109, 111-114, 120, 152, 186, 187

Fiber 5, 18, 26, 27, 33, 37, 40

G
Glycemic Index 6, 30, 34, 42, 184

H
Heart Attack 8, 13, 71, 116, 118-120, 188
Hypoglycemia 8, 93, 95-97, 99, 186

I
Immune system 24, 61, 113, 134, 139, 147, 151
Insulin 23, 30-32, 38-42, 45, 56, 59, 73, 74, 77, 95-97, 111, 117

K
Ketones 50, 58-60, 81

L
Leptin 6, 43, 45, 59

M
Monounsaturated fatty acids 5, 22

N
Neurotransmitters 7, 81-84, 86, 88, 89, 91, 93, 96, 97, 99, 129, 130

O
Obesity 2, 14, 25, 37-39, 42, 44, 45, 64, 76, 95, 102, 103, 119, 136, 155, 185

P
Polyunsaturated fats 5, 23

R
Recipes 10, 161, 163, 166, 192

S
Saturated Fats 5, 24, 25
Smoking 10, 117, 119, 129, 136, 157, 158, 190
Stress 8, 26, 84, 86, 90, 95, 96, 101-104, 106-109, 111-114, 124, 125, 129, 131, 133, 187

Sweet corn 6, 42
Symptoms 7, 8, 51, 64, 72, 91, 97, 104, 113, 119, 120, 124, 186, 188

T
Trans fat 5, 26
Treatment 7, 28, 66, 73, 90, 95, 153, 187

V
Vitamins 7, 9, 18, 22, 33, 37, 89-93, 99, 124, 125, 128, 131, 147, 150, 157-159, 188, 189

W
White flour 6, 39-41, 45
White pasta 6, 41, 45
White potatoes 6, 42
White rice 6, 32, 40, 41, 45, 185

About the Author

Tracy Ayton started her working life in the hair and beauty industry. While she loved this environment, she realized that mental health issues such as depression, apathy, anxiety, and weight issues were common. It didn't matter how good they looked; many of her customers were in trouble.

A bit of research convinced her that nutrition deficiencies were linked to these problems. She sold her beauty business, and embarked on a voyage of study and discovery. After completing nutrition studies, she put her research to work.

Tracy has worked with private clients and has worked at a medical center overseeing the nutritional care of patients with diabetes, weight management issues, and has assisted patients with fitness and disease prevention.

As she developed programs for clients, she realized there was a gap in the material available for those wanting to treat themselves, and this resulted in another career turn — to author.

Tracy was born in Kenya and subsequently moved to New Zealand where she completed her education and brought up a family. She lives and works in the Far North of New Zealand.

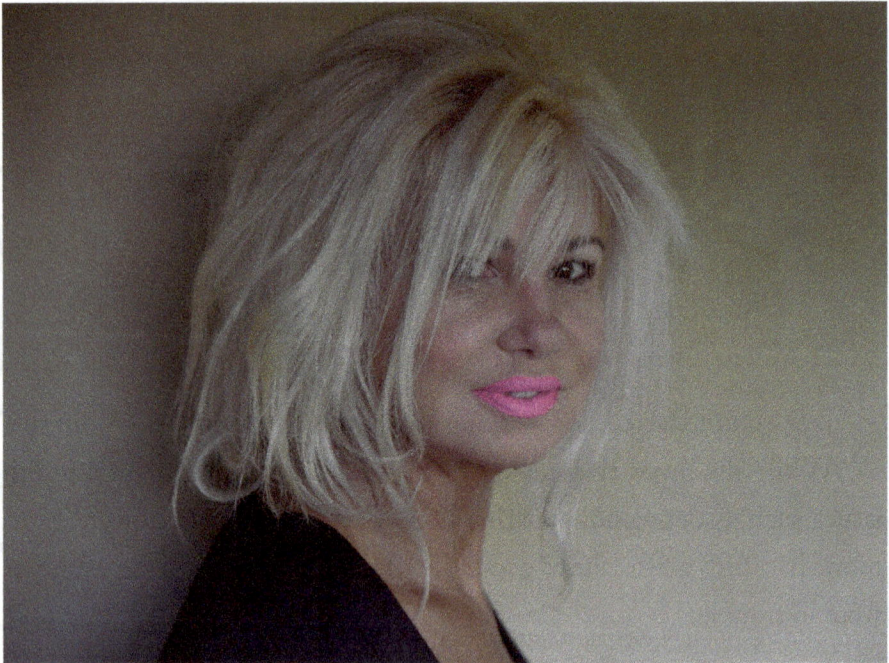

tracyayton.com • info@tracyayton.com